William K. Solberg/Glenn T. Clark, Temporomandibular Joint Problems

# Temporomandibular Joint Problems

## Biologic Diagnosis and Treatment


Edited by

William K. Solberg, D.D.S., M.S.D.
Professor and Chairman Section of Gnathology and Occlusion
Director, Temporomandibular and Facial Pain Clinic
School of Dentistry University of California at Los Angeles
Dental Research Institute, University of California

Glenn T. Clark, D.D.S., M.S.
Assistant Professor Section of Gnathology and Occlusion
Co-Director, Temporomandibular and Facial Pain Clinic
School of Dentistry University of California at Los Angeles



quintessence books

Quintessence Publishing Co., Inc. 1980
Chicago, Berlin, Rio de Janeiro and Tokyo

Second Printing

quintessence books



Lithography: Industrie- und Presseklischee, Berlin
Composition: Kupijai & Prochnow, Berlin
Printing and binding: North Central Publishing Co., St. Paul
Printed in U. S. A.

ISBN: 0-931386-18-7

# Proceedings of the 1st International Symposium, Newport Beach, California, February 22–24, 1979

The Department of Continuing Education in Health Sciences,
Division of Dentistry, UCLA Extension,
in Cooperation with the Newport Harbor Academy of Dentistry.

Organizing Committee

Symposium Chairman
William Solberg, D.D.S., M.S.D.
Chairman, Section of Gnathology and Occlusion
Director, Temporomandibular and Facial Pain Clinic
UCLA School of Dentistry

Local Arrangements Chairman
Carl Rieder, D.D.S.
Director, Newport Harbor Academy of Dentistry

Director, Continuing Education in Dentistry
UCLA Extension
Fredric Weissman, D.M.D.

*The objective of this book is to focus on the rapidly growing body of information about afflictions arising from disorders of the internal parts of the temporomandibular joint.*

# Table of Contents

# Contributors

Donald Blaschke, DDS
Assistant Professor, Section of Oral Radiology
Director, Maxillofacial Radiology Service
School of Dentistry, University of California
Los Angeles, California

Dr. Blaschke graduated from UCLA School of Dentistry in 1971, and later completed a residency in radiology at Vanderbilt University Hospital, Nashville, Tennessee. He is a fellow in the American Academy of Dental Radiology, and is an Assistant Attending Dentist at UCLA Hospital. Dr. Blaschke was among the first to successfully employ arthrography of the TMJ. In addition, Dr. Blaschke is conducting research on the radiographic determination of temporomandibular joint bony relationships; subsequent articles are forthcoming. Blaschke has five book chapters in preparation and in press; notably one entitled "Radiology" in a new volume by Sarnat and Laskin.

Tore Hansson, LDS, Odont. Dr.
Associate Professor of Stomatognathic Physiology and Dysfunction
School of Dentistry
University of Lund
Malmö, Sweden

Dr. Hansson graduated from the Royal Dental School, Malmö, Sweden, in 1969. He received his Doctor of Odontology from the University of Lund, Sweden in 1977. His thesis "Temporomandibular joint changes: occurence and development" has been a major contribution to the field of arthrology of the TMJ. Dr. Hansson has published two major articles on epidemiology of TMJ signs and symptoms and has been involved in correlating electromyographic and occlusal factors in patients with mandibular dysfunction. At present Dr. Hansson is a co-investigator on an extensive autopsy study being conducted at the Section of Gnathology, UCLA, which will attempt to identify and analyze the significance of TMJ changes in young adults.

Parker Mahan, DDS, Ph. D.
Professor and Chairman of the Department of Basic Dental Sciences
College of Dentistry,
University of Florida, Gainesville, Florida

Dr. Mahan graduated from the School of Dentistry, Emory University. He subsequently received his Ph. D. in physiology from the University of Rochester. Dr. Mahan is internationally known for his contributions in education and for over 50 research articles, which have been on head and neck pain, proprioception and occlusal function. He is a member of numerous professional and scientific societies and holds editorial positions with several journals. Dr. Mahan is co-editor with Dr. C. C. Alling of the book, *Facial Pain* published in 1977. He received the Jerome Schweitzer Research Award in 1976 from the Greater New York Academy of Prosthodontics. Dr. Mahan participates in a Pain Clinic at the University of Florida, specializing in facial and TMJ pain.

William McCarty, Jr., DMD
Diplomate of the American Board of Oral Surgery
Private practice limited to Oral and Maxillofacial Surgery
Montgomery, Alabama

Dr. McCarty is a consultant to the USAF, Wilford Hall, Lackland AFB, Texas. He has given numerous lectures on TMJ surgery and has performed over 500 cases of TMJ surgery. He is a fellow of the Academy of Craniomandibular Disorders. Dr. McCarty, in collaboration with Dr. William Farrar, is particularly recognized for developing the diagnostic rationale for conservative arthroplasties in treating internal derangements of the TMJ.

Willy Krogh-Poulsen, LDS, Odont. Dr. h. c.
Professor and formerly Head of the Department of Stomatognathic Physiology and Dysfunction
Royal Dental College
Copenhagen, Denmark

Dr. Krogh-Poulsen recently stepped down from a long and impressive career in dental education. He is a pioneer and international leader in the area of mandibular function and dysfunction. His ideas and expertise on the clinical management of occlusal problems have had a dramatic impact on educators and clinicians throughout the world. Particularly, Dr. Krogh-Poulsen is recognized for his contributions in the area of pedagogy and curriculum development in the field of occlusion. Professor Krogh-Poulsen has been the editor and author of several books and articles on prosthetics, dental anatomy and stomatognathic physiology. His most important recent work has been as chief editor of a unique textbook on stomatognathic physiology and dysfunction for use in Scandinavia.

Daniel Laskin, DDS, MS
Professor and Head of the Department of Oral and Maxillofacial Surgery
College of Dentistry
Director of the Temporomandibular Joint and Facial
Pain Research Center University of Illinois Medical Center
Deputy Chairman of the Division of Oral Surgery,
Cook County Hospital
Chicago, Illinois

Dr. Laskin received his DDS degree from Indiana University School of Dentistry and his Master of Science degree at the University of Illinois. He is a Diplomate of the American Board of Oral and Maxillofacial Surgery and has served on its Advisory Committee. He is Past President of the American Association of Oral and Maxillofacial Surgeons, and is editor of their AAOMS Forum. He is also editor of the Journal of Oral Surgery. He is a member of Omicron Kappa Upsilon, Sigma Xi and a Fellow of both the American and International College of Dentists. Dr. Laskin has made over 300 contributions to the literature in the field of Oral Surgery and in Dental Research. In 1978 he received the American Association of Oral and Maxillofacial Surgeons Research Recognition Award. Dr. Laskin is the co-author of two major books about to be published, one on the TMJ and the other on oral and maxillofacial surgery.

Benjamin Moffett, Ph. D.
Professor of Orthodontics
University of Washington, Dental Faculty

Dr. Moffett received his B. A. from Syracuse University and his Ph. D. from New York University. He has been a Visiting Professor at the University of Nijmegen (the Netherlands) and at the Medical University of So. Carolina. Dr. Moffett has published over 35 articles on various aspects of bones and joints of the craniofacial complex, including his much cited 1964 publication on articular remodeling in the adult TMJ. Recently Dr. Moffett has been involved in the management of patients in the TMJ Clinic at the University of Washington and in the process has applied his expertise in clinical anatomy and physiology for developing systems of diagnosis of TMJ afflictions.

Torsten Öberg, LDS, Odont. Dr.
Professor and Chairman of the Department of
Stomatognathic Physiology and Dysfunction,
School of Dentistry
University of Lund, Malmö, Sweden

Professor Öberg received his degree in dentistry from the Royal School of Dentistry, Stockholm. He received his Doctor of Odontology from the University of Umeå, Sweden. Dr. Öberg is a member of many European dental societies. Dr. Öberg is head of the same department once chaired by Ulf Posselt, and has continued to develop this department so as to maintain its international notoriety. Dr. Öberg's research and clinical investigations have been on the anatomy and pathology of the TMJ in various animal models and in humans. In these investigations he has frequently utilized radiology as a research tool. He has published over 35 articles and book chapters, and is considered a world expert in the area of radiology and pathology of the temporomandibular joint.

# Preface

The objective of this Symposium was to expose and evaluate the rapidly growing body of information about afflictions arising from disorders within the temporomandibular joint (TMJ). It was the task of each speaker at this symposium to focus on this objective. Other important aspects of TMJ dysfunction such as the role of the neuromuscular system were not discussed prominently. Specifically, the international panel was selected to discuss the significance of new findings about TMJ function, radiology, arthrography, internal derangements, remodeling and osteoarthrosis. To consider the possibility that previously unrecognized problems within the TMJ articulation might contribute in a major way to the production of symptoms of the so-called TMJ syndrome was the major impetus for organizing this gathering.

A most pleasant occasion for this Symposium was to honor Professor *Willy G. Krogh-Poulsen,* who has recently retired from his position as professor of the Department of Stomatognathic Physiology and Dysfunction at the Royal Dental College, Copenhagen, Denmark. Dr. *Krogh-Poulsen* continues his life-long career as an educator and scholar which has earned him an international reputation as a foremost pioneer in the education of students, clinicians and researchers in the field of stomatognathic dysfunction. It is with the greatest pleasure and gratitude that we dedicate this book to Professor *Willy Krogh-Poulsen.*

We wish to thank Dr. *Carl Rieder,* and selected members of the Newport Harbor Academy of Dentistry for their expertise and careful attention to detail that made the Symposium a splendid affair. We are grateful to Dr. Fredric Weissman and his staff from University Extension, UCLA, for their efforts in promotion and administration. The Word Processing Center, Dental Illustration and Dental Photography, UCLA School of Dentistry receive our thanks for their cooperation in producing the manuscript. We are indebted to Drs. Mary Penn and Karen Gjerde for their editorial assistance.

We are especially grateful to the speakers who, despite extremely involved schedules, were willing to join with us for the documentation of the evidence and for the subsequent discussion of the issues which took place. The chapters in this volume were taken from transcriptions of the Symposium which every speaker revised for publication. For their generosity and promptness in completing this important task, we owe the speakers a large measure of gratitute. Ample time was given to discussion by the speakers and to questions from the audience, which are also published in edited form. During the final stages of publication we learned with great regret of the death of Professor *Torsten Öberg* on January 22, 1980. Dr. *Öberg's* untimely passing is surely a great loss for those who have been graced by his warmth, optimism and dignity. Dr. *Öberg's* fundamental studies on the arthrology of the temporomandibular joint will continue to symbolize his vital presence—aiding those taking up future challenging aspects of temporomandibular pain and dysfunction.

The Editors
William K. Solberg/Glenn T. Clark

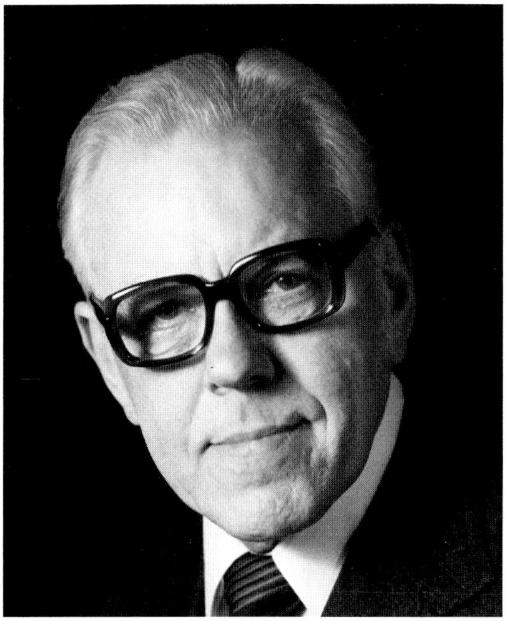

# Dedication

Professor Willy G. Krogh-Poulsen

"The first time I saw *Willy Krogh-Poulsen* was many years ago as a student at the Royal Dental College Copenhagen. We were all sitting in the auditorium, the room was in an uproar and the noise of the crowd deafening. Suddenly a breeze of silence came over the auditorium as someone said 'He's on his way.' The door opened and the professor entered in his long white gown, followed by his assistant and secretary, like solemn bodyguards. He went to the podium and at a nod of his head, all the students sat down, silent. As he spoke, the charisma of this man, his reputation, his knowledge and his experience made us want to absorb his every word.

*Willy Krogh-Poulsen* devoted his life to education as a full Professor of Prosthodontics. He developed the Department of Stomatognathic Physiology and Dysfunction, which has become a model throughout the world. He has had always one goal, which he passed on to us in his last lecture to the student body and faculty of the Royal Dental College at Copenhagen in September 1977, 'Let us try to make it easier for those people who have problems. Let their lives be acceptable and tolerable, and if not, let us find the reason and then take proper action.'

Ladies and Gentlemen, would you join me in greeting our respected mentor, Professor *Willy Krogh-Poulsen.*"

Introductory remarks by Dr. *Knud Flygenring*, Class of 1960, Royal Dental College, Copenhagen, Denmark.

# From Occlusion Theory to Oral Physiotherapy

by W. Krogh-Poulsen*

*Almost everything which man undertakes within a society is, in the deepest sense, aimed at an effort to make life acceptable for humanity; or to fathom why it is not, and in such cases, to take the necessary precautions or measures.* An important element in this context is the level of health of the individual, the group, and society. The World Health Organization has pointed out that health does not mean only the absence of illness; health also manifests itself as a sense of well-being not merely somatic but also psychic and social, i. e. by balance in the relationships to one's surroundings. This is intensely experienced by those who work with patients having malfunctions in the masticatory system and its co-functioning structures, and who suffer from the resulting disorders. In such patients the somatic, psychic or social factors can be out of harmony, and the interaction between them may no longer function at an optimum level. The ordinary sense of well-being is lost.

## Character of the condition

These patients may have persistent or repetitive pain or discomfort of the face, maxillae, temporomandibular joints, head, throat, or neck. Other examples of somatic discomfort are tenderness or fatigue in the muscles, pain or difficulty with chewing or with certain movements of the lower jaw, soreness of the teeth, reduced ability to open the mouth, and cracking or crepitation of the temporomandibular joints. Oral malfunctions can also be accompanied by a feeling of globulus (a lump in the throat) or other unusual oropharyngeal sensations.

The symptom of cracking (clicking or popping) occurs very frequently, most often in a form tolerated by the patient. In some patients, however, the malfunction in the jaw joint makes the cracking sound audible for others. In such a case, a social problem may arise; namely, if the symptom attracts the attention of others while dining and becomes an annoyance to them. Symptoms of the above mentioned type are, for some people, so slight or sporadic that they are ignored. In others, they can be so serious that they cause a reduction in working abilities and related social complications of an economic and communicative nature.

Pain, as in a headache, can usually be tolerated in the case of a single attack but if the condition repeats itself on a daily basis, the individual's condition may be affected and expressed by feelings of irritation with family members, fellow workers or others. Such irritation may convert to anxiety or uneasiness, especially if the cause for the problem is not understood and no relief is

* In 1977 Professor Krogh-Poulsen retired from 42 years of teaching at the Royal Dental College, Copenhagen. This article is a translation from Danish of his last official lecture, which was first published in Tandlägebladet, 82:125–128, 1978.

presented. In this manner the condition comes to affect the patient psychologically.

Even if dentists usually have an understanding of this type of patient and his problems, much remains to be done regarding the recognition of this patient group, interpretation of the symptoms and findings, and interest in the treatment of such patients. It is, therefore, an important assignment for dentistry to achieve full competence of the profession in this area.

## The dimensions of the problem

Epidemiological examinations have given us a good understanding of the frequency of function-related illness in the masticatory system within Scandinavia; and the situation will probably be similar in other areas of the world.

Approximately one-half of all people have one or more of the above mentioned symptoms. The symptoms are present in all age groups from 5—6 year-olds on up in every social class and in both sexes. Most reports find an excess of women with these symptoms. However, other epidemiologists have reported a more even distribution. It will be one of the assignments of future researchers to account for the causal relationships and other biological and social factors which might influence the sex distribution, and possibly give us an explanation for this peculiarity.

The occurrence of dysfunction of the masticatory system is so frequent that patients of this type are present in every dentist's practice. However, many patients are not recognized because their symptoms are subliminal. That is to say, their discomfort is so small that a need for treatment has not become manifest. Even if only a small portion of the patients have a condition which actually demands treatment, the frequent occurence of patients with function-related problems implies that a significant portion of diagnosis and treatment of this patient group must necessarily be executed by the practicing dentist. Both pre and post-graduate education in this area must, therefore, receive high priority in order to insure the population an adequate treatment service.

The problem is one of urgency. To solve it will place demands upon both the public and the private sectors of health care and call for more manpower. In this connection it is important to be alert to the relationship between the actual need for treatment and the patient's request for help. Such needs or requests do not develop simultaneously or at the same tempo, since they are dependent on different factors.

## Prophylaxis

As time goes on it becomes more and more evident to those who are working with this condition that one cannot "treat oneself out of the problem", but must work up to and solve it through the use of prophylactic measures as in other types of odontological prophylaxis.

Until further research supplies us with other tools, prophylaxis must be seen as containing two significant aspects, both of which are related to the dentist's activities; in addition, it must be recognized that function-related suffering is frequently iatrogenically determined.

The first aspect of prophylaxis is encompassed in the expression, "respect for nature". The morphology of the natural occlusal surfaces must serve as the model when artificial restoration is undertaken or occlusal surfaces are remodeled by grinding, so that supracontacts or interferences are avoided. Nature takes her revenge against those who go against her, here as in other realms. In occlusal rehabilitation, functional occlusal waxing can assure optimal and interference free occlusal contact relationships, both in the intercuspal position and when the mandible follows its natural pattern of movement.

The second aspect of prophylaxis concerns tooth extraction. Reluctance in the decision of removing teeth is necessary, especially if the intention is only to alter the hygienic status of the mouth. The migration and tilting of the neighboring teeth which follows extraction is a frequent cause of occlusal interferences and the resulting damage can be worse than that which was the primary cause for surgical intervention. Regular control of the remaining dentition with special attention given to the position of the neighboring teeth is therefore an important prophylactic factor.

All prophylaxis acts by intervention into the origin and/or developmental mechanism of the pathologic/pathogenic complex. Therefore, a detailed knowledge of the etiology, pathogenesis and initial clinical symptoms of function-related disorders is of great importance. In this area, we know a great deal today, but far from enough, and intensive research is also necessary on this front.

## The pathological response

Function-related disorders are localized, as a whole, to structures in the locomotor system, especially to the muscles and their tendinous attachments as well as the structures of the joints. The locomotor system also includes the masticatory system. An understanding of the specific nature of the function-related disorders in the masticatory system therefore presupposes a general knowledge of the characteristics and activities of the neuromuscular system as well as the response to work, exertion, and strain of the locomotor system under acceptable functioning situations. Thus, the approach of work-physiology has to be included in the field of research on the function of the masticatory system.

When a certain outer or inner limit of influence is exceeded, the masticatory system works under conditions which may become intolerable over a longer period of time. In such cases, the etiological and pathogenic problems correspond directly to those for which the physiotherapist treats other parts of the locomotor system.

In this context, the study of the nature and the location of the boundary between tolerable and intolerable functional conditions plays an important role, since function-related disorders occur under intolerable activity in structures which are involved in a given function. Most often the intolerable activity implies forces working over a long period of time with high intensity. As a result, the structures in the exposed portion of the system become the object of prolonged traumatization. An example of this is the lengthy, powerful tension that can arise in the elevator muscles of the mandible as well as in its protractor and laterotractor muscles during clenching and grinding. Also, extreme unguarded movements or activity in unaccustomed positions, can cause a pathological response in the involved tissues.

The response to such continuing "microtraumatic" influences varies for the different tissue types. Some of the most common examples are myofascitis, traction periostitis, or osteoarthrosis with structural changes in the soft tissues, exostosis or cystic changes in the osseous structure. The common trait in such reactions is that they always appear in connective tissues or in mesodermal-derived structures. For example, we perceive myofascitis as an aseptic, inflammatory reaction in the muscle's interstitial connective tissue. The changes referred to in the articular structures behave in a similar manner, with the modifications caused by localization and tissue types as previously mentioned.

The principle of development of pathological tissue reaction is known in part, but on the cellular level the processes remain unclear. Therefore research in connective tissue behavior must become a part of future studies within this subject area.

An understanding of how the microtraumatic activity originates is in the process of development through electromyographic and other neurophysiologic techniques. But there are still many unanswered questions of relevance, an example being the relationship between supracontracts and muscular hyperactivity. Here too, then, are fields which must be looked into in the near future.

## Examination and diagnostics

For the patients, in the meantime, the crucial problem is to be helped, and in the course of the last 10—15 years a rational method of clinical examination has been established. This leads to a rational diagnosis which encompasses the tissue lesions as well as the malfunction and underlying general factors, including the level of psychomotor activity. The result is a rational and relatively simple therapy.

The characteristic feature of the method developed in our department for examination, diagnosis, and treatment is that it has been possible to abandon time and resource-demanding procedures, consciously emphasizing methods which can be put into effect in general practice, thus enabling the practicing dentist to participate in the recognition, evaluation and treatment of the function-related disorders.

The examination places its primary focus on disclosing signs of malfunction due to unconscious hyperactivity in the lower jaw's system of movement and in the co-functional structures. At the same time the possibilities of mandibular movement and the occlusal contact relationships are elucidated with the goal of uncovering and verifying the symptom provoking contacts or activities.

The case history and the information from conversations with the patient are a significant part of the examination, because this often leads to a better understanding of the many factors which can contribute to the emergency and course of the disorder.

The diagnostic procedure evaluates findings and information in reference to (a) the localization and the nature of the symptom provoking tissue lesion, (b) the specific malfunction which has induced the pathological tissue reaction, and (c) the possible general condition which lies behind the malfunction and reaction pattern.

Differential diagnostic considerations often demand broad diagnostic knowledge in the odontological and especially the related medical areas. In this respect a considerable intensification of clinical research and an expansion of the theoretical foundation is needed.

## Treatment

The treatment is goal oriented and for the most part quite simple. Mainly it aims at suppressing the exaggerated muscular activity:

– *generally* by lowering the level of the patient's psychomotor activity through explanation and counseling, and in some cases through the administration of psychoactive drugs for a brief period;
– *specifically* by correcting the malfunction and alleviating its direct effects, especially by establishing mandibular stabilization through multipoint occlusal contacts. This causes a change in the afferent nerve impulse pattern, which is initiated by the occlusal supracontacts the result being a reduction of the habitual, muscular activity.
In most cases the stabilization of the mandible is primarily established by occlusal splints and later followed up through occlusal adjustment by grinding or occlusal reconstruction.
Additional treatment of the muscular tension can be obtained through the help of behavior modification, while the pathological tissue response in muscles and joints may be treated with physiotherapy.
We are facing a new dimension in dentistry and an increase in our inter-relationship with medicine (rheumatology, neurology and clinical psychology) must be anticipated. Through this, a specialty area will develop so that it will become, what in fact it already is: *oral physiotherapy.*

## The course of development

In progressing towards the present state of the subject, there have been laborious efforts and lifelong contributions from a long chain of clinicians and research specialists. Without forgetting the many who worked in silence, or those whose contributions have never been praised, I would like to mention a few individuals.
*Bonwill, Carl Christensen, Gysi* and *McCollum* laid the ground work, between 1850 and 1930, to all of the presently known methods of treatment which aim at establishing a tolerable, artificial occlusion whether it concerns grinding, bridges, or removable prosthetics. They achieved this by establishing even, gliding occlusal contact and by establishing an occlusion which could stabilize the lower jaw against the cranium in every contact situation.
Others, *Kawamura* and *Møller* for example, are more interested in the neuromuscular activities of the masticatory system under normal conditions. Their contributions have given us a background for understanding the nature of pathological functions.
A third group, among them *Karolyi* and *Posselt,* concentrated on the study of different function-related processes and the possible pathology resulting from them. Focus was primarily on the problems concerning bruxism and the resulting tissue damage in the periodontium and temporomandibular joints. They were quick to acknowledge that this area concerns a patient group requiring special attention. Posselt, especially, saw the challenge and took it up and the rest of us have, to the best of our abilities, followed in his and the other leaders' footsteps.
All of these odontologists have commonly acknowledged their patient's need for help, and each in his own way sought to solve a portion of these problems. They have lived up to something which is fundamental in every medical person's attitude, namely, that he – consciously or unconsciously – attempts to follow the line I stated in the introduction: *to make life acceptable to humanity; or to fathom why it is not, and in such cases, to take the necessary precautions or measures.*
With this the ring is closed and the directional arrow pointed. All I have left to say is thank you for all of the years and I wish you luck in the future.

# I. Classification and Diagnosis of Temporomandibular Joint Disturbances

by Benjamin Moffett

It is a joy to be with friends and colleagues having a common interest in the subject to be discussed during the next two days, and it is especially enjoyable to have a format arranged by Dr. *Solberg* and his colleagues that allows for maximum exchange of ideas. In the few comments that I will present to open the Symposium, my intent is not to give complete coverage to the topic assigned to me. In fact, it has already been determined that we should focus our presentations and discussions on those aspects of TMJ problems that involve the joint specifically, both its structure and its function. Therefore, I will restrict my comments on diagnostic approach to those aspects. By so doing, I do not imply that there isn't a broader or more far-ranging area to be covered in a comprehensive approach to TMJ diagnosis. I must acknowledge, first of all, that the information to be discussed today is derived from the work of my clinical colleagues, Dr. *Stephen Teel*, Dr. *Kenneth Morrison* and other members of the dental faculty. We owe thanks to many other individuals at the Medical Center in Seattle, whose services we have had to call upon frequently for diagnostic and treatment assistance in identifying the problems of a given patient.

Because I am to review briefly the classification and diagnosis of these problems, I will quote an introductory passage from the *Manual of International Statistical Classification of Diseases, Injuries and Causes of Death (MISCD), 1967:* "There are many approaches to the classification of disease. The anatomist, for example, may desire a classification based on the part of the body affected. The pathologist, on the other hand, is primarily interested in the nature of the disease process. The clinician must consider disease from these two angles, but needs further knowledge of etiology." Having left anatomy some 20 years ago in order to work in the clinical milieu, I certainly would identify myself in the third category.

The manual just referred to is helpful in that it shows how our colleagues in medicine describe the kinds of clinical problems with which they are confronted. This international classification of diseases is organized according to the organ systems, and in Part 13 it deals with diseases of the musculoskeletal system and connective tissue. Here we can find time-tested terms; diagnostic labels that our medical colleagues apply to problems involving articulations. In this manual there is a different kind of terminology, more biologically oriented, than the labels we use in the dental literature for TMJ problems. If we look at page 226 from that guide we see, under the heading of internal derangements of joints, some concepts and terminology that are applicable to the temporomandibular joint. This section identifies such problems in menisci as degeneration, rupture, and tears. Later, on the manual lists other injuries such as dislocations, sprains, strains, loose bodies or cartilages in the joint. I see no reason why we should not include such findings in our diagnostic approach to the TMJ, a structure that is basically a synovial joint.

In regard to other joints which also have discs, physicians talk about prolapse, protrusion, rupture and herniation of intervertebral discs. For the various articulations throughout this manual we see diagnostic labels that illustrate how we might interpret symptoms in the TMJ.

In our attempts to classify TMJ problems, perhaps first we should define the term, diagnosis. I like the comment in a book by Logan Clendening, the late medical diagnostician, where diagnosis is defined by Webster as determining the nature of a disease. That "a" is important. We are dealing with **a** single instance, **a** single individual and his disease. No generalizations are involved. I think that's a good point to keep in mind, because it is evident from the clinical literature on TMJ problems that many of the diagnostic concepts or labels used there are based on generalizations and tend to lose sight of that particular individual who has just walked through the door with a specific set of symptoms. Clendening stresses that diagnosis is the application of the data of science to a specific case. I wish to enlarge on that point by strongly refuting the misconception that there is a difference between a clinician and a researcher. A clinician must be a researcher by the nature of his work. The dialogue that goes on between the clinician and the patient must obey the same principles of methodology as the dialogue that goes on in the laboratory between the nonclinical researcher and the subject of his investigation. Diagnosis is the process of formulating a hypothesis and testing the validity of that hypothesis with a treatment plan that allows you to document the patient's responses to treatment. *George Bernard Shaw* comments that diagnosis ought to mean the finding out of all that is wrong with a particular patient and why. These guidelines from Clendening and Shaw seem to have been ignored in regard to TMJ problems.

I was alarmed recently to discover how much these principles of diagnostic methodology are neglected even by those responsible for determining the objectives of dental research. Last year I submitted a research proposal to the National Institute of Dental Research based on data and concepts derived from a seven-year study of *all* TMJ patients appearing at our research clinic. The proposal was for a multidisciplinary approach to diagnosis based on identifying a problem list for each individual patient and developing from that an appropriately individualized treatment plan. This was proposed as a substitute for the currently popular syndromal approach. The proposal was the most thoroughly prepared and documented application of all those that I have submitted over the past 25 years. Nevertheless, the Study Section for Oral Biology and Medicine perfunctorily rejected it without further discussion and without a site visit to examine our clinic and its data. The reasons given for this rejection deny the interest in and need for this very symposium. The study section concluded, without allowing a challenge of their reasons, that the proposed diagnostic methodology applied to TMJ patients was an "overkill" and that, in their opinion, the present approach is adequate for treating such patients. This combination of ignorance and dogma is inexcusable in a so-called peer review process but it illustrates the magnitude of the conceptual problem that we face.

After thinking critically about our present

approach to diagnosis, I would characterize it as our biggest single obstacle to the successful management of TMJ problems. A diagnostic approach that is useful at one point in time can later become an obstacle to progress when it creates a diagnostic label that restricts our ability to think further. Words become a prison when we accept and cling to them uncritically in a field that is far from conceptual and clinical perfection. The way we think in arriving at a diagnosis must follow scientific principles. Regardless of whatever else the scientific method may be, it must be logical and *self-critical.* We can only think with words and those words must be challenged continually as our base of knowledge and our perspectives grow.

The difficulties that TMJ patients have in finding successful treatment originate in our diagnostic inadequacies, not in the complexities of the biologic system confronting us. After studying the developmental, aging and pathologic changes that occur in TMJs from conception to death, I can assure you that this joint obeys the same biologic laws as do all articulations and their associated musculoskeletal components. Throughout its life cycle the TMJ displays shifting equilibria between changes in form and changes in function, just as all joints do. In trying to identify and analyze these shifts, it seems to me that we are our own worst enemies. Instead of focusing a diagnostic label on the problems of an individual patient, we have adopted a basket label, erroneously called a syndrome, that we apply uncritically to a large group of patients with differing and multiple problems. This is a serious obstacle because when we label something a syndrome of pain and dysfunction, we explain nothing. We do not identify any underlying biologic or pathologic processes, we deny that there are associated morphologic alterations to be treated, and we proceed then to rely on a symptom-oriented treatment formula applied indiscriminately to all patients placed in that diagnostic basket. The time has come for us to develop a set of more precise, explanatory labels for the variety of TMJ problems confronting us. The clinical evidence to be presented at this symposium will surely give us the opportunity to improve our labels provided our minds are prepared to do so.

If you will accept Clendening's view that our diagnostic task is to determine the nature of a patient's disease, we should now define the term, disease. I like the definition used in *Gould's Medical Dictionary* (1972) because it takes us back to the underlying biologic processes. Disease is a response to injury, sickness or illness — a failure of the adaptive mechanism of an organism to counteract adequately the stimuli or stresses to which it is subject, resulting in a disturbance in function or structure of any part.

After studying the adaptive responses of different articulations, I would say that we will not find much of a disturbance in function without having a corresponding degree of alteration in structure. The interplay between form and function is so inseparable, that the problem which we label in the clinical literature as being a dysfunction, inevitably has a corresponding degree of alteration in form. Dysmorphology goes hand-in-hand with dysfunction, and we must be prepared conceptually to recognize the existence of these parallel changes in patients coming to us for the diagnosis of possible disturbances in function and structure of the TMJ and its associated components.

If we accept the idea that the disease is a response to some stimulus, the stimuli causing these clinical responses have to be identified by a careful history that requires as much time as does the clinical examination (Fig. 1). To the extent that we can document the stimuli and responses, we then proceed to modify them clinically in some beneficial way focusing as much of the treatment plan on the stimuli or the etiologic factors as we do on the patient's disease responses. We probably are not going to get a lasting resolution of a problem if we don't attempt to deal with etiologic factors. Treatment of symptoms alone may help to identify a tentative diagnosis, but this certainly isn't the end point towards which we are reaching.

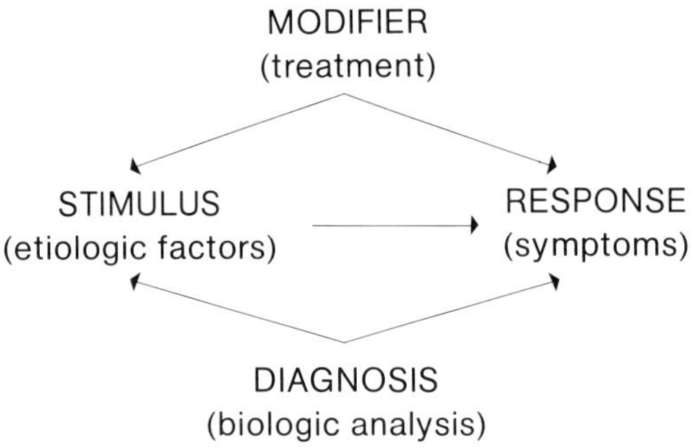


Fig. 1

At some point in developing the treatment plan we must attempt to explain what we think is behind these clinical responses and identify, if possible, the causative stimuli. Then we must state this analysis in words that indicate the biologic or pathologic processes that created the patient's symptoms. This verbal explanation can be made after we have tested our hypothesis and validated it or we can do it intuitively at the beginning. In either case, the diagnosis ought to be an etiologic explanation of the clinical symptoms stated in biologic or pathologic terms. Good diagnostic labels will provide an explanation to the extent that knowledge allows us to do so. To verbalize a diagnosis as pain or dysfunction is not making anybody wiser. We want to get beneath the symptoms of pain and dysfunction, to identify *what* is in a state of dysfunction, and then use a diagnostic label to explain why by indicating what the cause and effect relationships might be.

A logical way to do this is to list after the detailed examination and history each patient's problems, remembering that suspected stimuli or etiologic factors should be included as part of the problem. In a problem list we identify everything we have learned so far about the etiologic factors along with the patient's clinical responses. We don't list these in any specific order and we don't express them in diagnostic terms because a problem list isn't intended to be a diagnostic analysis. We are not paying much attention at this step to cause and effect relationships. We want merely to identify, at a symptomatic level, *all* the problems with which we must help the patient cope. Later we will try to put it into the context of a diagnostic explanation.

Usually there are at least three or four problem entries in each patient's chart, and we state them in plain English: popping noises, grating noises, two kinds of joint pain (inflammatory and instantaneous), muscle pain, dislocation, catching or locking, etc. In listing the problems that apply, we don't distinguish between clinical responses and etiologic factors — they both must be dealt with. We include clenching habits, unusual sleeping positions, a history of specific kinds of trauma, personality characteristics that might be involved, unusual kinds of stress, other health problems, occlusal aspects such as open bite, centric and balancing interferences, radiographic changes, the nature of the patient's response to the clinician as he tries to identify the problems, facial growth patterns, adverse effects from previous treatments, and whether or not the complaints of the patient seem clinically logical or illogical.

And then, what do you do with such a problem list? It has several important functions. First, it provides a baseline from which to evaluate the patient's future responses to treatment. Does the problem list change as treatment proceeds? Which problems are diminishing — which are worse? Second, by relating the problem list to the time of initial onset of the patient's disease, we learn how TMJ diseases evolve sequentially through different stages. There are two ways to accomplish this. Some patients with long-standing TMJ symptoms can well describe the sequence in which their symptoms arose and were in turn replaced by other symptoms as their diseases evolved. The other method for gaining such insights is to look at a large sample of patients cross-sectionally, thus establishing a symptom profile for diseases of recent onset as contrasted with those of long duration. Both techniques allow the clinician to recognize that a seemingly insignificant symptom, such as a clicking joint, usually gives a warning that, if untreated, the joint will later develop more serious symptoms of instantaneous joint pain, catching, locking and grating noise or crepitus. This symptom chain is a definite trend in a sample of TMJ patients documented by the problem list approach. Once the trend has been established with such data, it allows you to recognize the incompetence of those individuals who would have us believe that a clicking TMJ is of no clinical significance and need not be considered in designing a treatment plan. When this kind of insight emerges, the problem list approach tells you that your treatment plan must be expanded to deal with a problem previously thought to be insignificant.

There are many parallels of this type of learning to be gained from sequential problem lists. For instance, the most fundamental insight to emerge is recognizing the pattern of how TMJ diseases evolve over time. The first symptoms to appear clinically are those of dysfunction. Invariably the clinical signs of morphologic alterations are not seen until later on in the course of the worsening disease. However, the apparent time lag between the onset of dysfunction and the appearance of morphologic changes disappears when a histologic study is made of TMJ specimens obtained at surgery and autopsy. Furthermore, biologic principles would lead one to conclude that these changes occur hand in hand.

A disease of recent onset becomes labeled as a dysfunction only because it is easier to clinically detect the signs of dysfunction at that stage. However, to give it such a diagnostic label is a conceptual artifact, an error that in turn creates an inadequate treatment plan — one that doesn't include morphologic repair at an early stage in the evolving disease. Perforated discs remain unrepaired surgically or removed instead of being restored because the superficial diagnostic label of TMJ dysfunction channels our thinking away from treatment plans aimed at morphologic repair and regeneration.

I would like to expand these specific illustrations of evolving diseases into a schematic spectrum of clinical disease responses that we recognize first as signs of dysfunction and only later as morphologic alterations (Table I). The time interval between the clinical recognition of these two types of symptoms will diminish as we employ additional diagnostic techniques aimed at visualizing the nonmineralized articular tissues. The earliest morphologic changes in joint diseases occur in the capsule, menisci and articular tissues of synovial joints. It is very exciting, therefore, to see that TMJ arthrography is one of the main themes to be discussed in this program.

Because it will take time for the necessary changes to occur in our conceptual

**Table I** Clinical disease responses

| | | |
|---|---|---|
| **Dysfunction** ← | → | **Morphologic Alterations** |
| ↑ | **Treatment procedures** | ↑ |
| **Modify Behavior** | | **Stimulate Repair** |
| Occlusal modification | | Surgery |
| Training | | Rest |
| Biofeedback | | Medication |
| Counseling | | Occlusal modification |
| Medication | | **Prosthesis** |
| | | Skeletal |
| | | Dental |

**Table II** Responses of 52 patients* to occlusal splint therapy (2 months to over 1 year post treatment)

| Response | Patients with occlusal interferences | Patients without occlusal interferences |
|---|---|---|
| Major Improvement | 22 } – 80% | 11 } – 80% |
| Minor Improvement | 8 | 1 |
| Unchanged | 7 | 3 |
| Total | 37 | 15 |

approach to diagnosis, we will continue to base early treatment on plans aimed at the dysfunctional aspects of TMJ diseases. The correction of dysfunction implies that jaw behavior will be changed and, in fact, the initial treatment modalities modify jaw behavior. Preliminary data show, for instance, that occlusal splints reduce the muscle symptoms of jaw dysfunction equally well in TMJ patients with and without significant occlusal discrepancies (Table II).

Our present diagnostic inadequacies result in a postponement of the treatment modalities aimed at correcting morphologic

* Splints used on 58 out of 114 patients. No response data available on 6 splint patients.

alterations in the TMJ until advanced destruction has occurred. In fact, most of the surgical treatment plans presently used for TMJ problems aim at removing parts of the destroyed joint instead of intercepting early deterioration with procedures aimed at stimulating biologic repair and remodeling.
Unfortunately, my time is running short, so I'll conclude these remarks that are aimed at principles of diagnostic methodology by acknowledging in advance the material to be presented by the remaining speakers on the program. They will document in great detail the kinds of morphologic alterations being ignored in our current approach to diagnosis and will also propose appropriate treatment procedures for intercepting early structural changes. I hope that my comments will provide a basis for discussion. Please do not regard them as a comprehensive approach to TMJ diagnosis, but as one that is focused upon so-called internal derangements in this joint.

## Discussion

Discussant: Willy Krogh-Poulsen

I would like to comment first on some ideas about the diagnosis or the diagnostic procedure that came up here. First of all, what we are discussing here are classifications of reactions to biomechanical stresses. We are not talking about infection, or macrotrauma, or tumors. In so doing we can set up a scheme very much similar to that which Dr. *Moffett* has talked about and which we could use in our teaching. When we examine a patient we observe the signs and symptoms. From that information we try to describe the structural changes which cause the signs and symptoms. But in order to find out how we can indirectly treat the structural changes, for example by changing the occlusion with splints or grinding, we have to isolate the dysfunction. So after the structural diagnosis we consider a dysfunctional diagnosis. What is going on in the joint is always connected with the supply of energy to the joint in one way or another. Muscular energy can be concentrated in the joint structure, for example directly through the pull of the lateral pterygoid muscle or indirectly over the occlusal joint (to use Dr. *Moffett's* term) in pressing or bruxing. Observation and deduction together will provide the dysfunctional diagnosis. This will tell us how we have to bring these distorted structures to peace so there may be natural tissue repair, and a normalization of the dysfunction. Therefore, the dysfunction diagnosis is so very important.
Behind the dysfunction diagnosis, there is a third layer of diagnosis which we have to recognize, and that is what I call the psychomotoric activity level. The psychomotoric activity level was also touched upon by Dr. *Moffett,* when he pointed out the influence of stress in daily life or things which are boring to the patient or his communication with other people. Psychic and social problems are involved at this level and give the general stimulus for muscular activity. We have found that if we structure our description of the situation in this way, it is much easier to find out how to treat the patient in order to change the dysfunction into natural function and so let nature do its work on the structural disorders.
I would also like to comment about the location of the pathological response. To me it doesn't matter whether a patient's responses are seen in muscles, in tendons, in joint structures, in hard dental tissues, or in

periodontal ligaments. The response can appear in all of the tissues in the stomatognathic system. We are concentrating on the joint today, but in our patients we will find the responses all over. In trying to analyze the situations in the patient, I have found that the tissue response will always be located in the area of the largest concentration of energy. That is, where the forces are concentrated over a long period of time and where we have a high level of concentrated energy at a specific point, we will have a pathologic tissue response. This is exactly what Dr. *Moffett* showed us—when there is a high concentration of energy in the joint, structural changes occurred which could result in total destruction of the joint. Now, regarding the dysfunctional activity, we can observe where this point of energy is and consider how to dissipate this concentration. This is exactly what we do when we modify the occlusal scheme since the muscular energy will spread when you equilibrate the occlusion. We have observed that Class II orthodontic patients are more prone to have pathologic conditions in their muscles or in the joint structures. We have made clinical observations that these patients often are working their mandibles more forward or sometimes just resting their mandibles on the incisal edges or grinding a little there. This is only possible if the lateral pterygoid muscle is working over a long period of time and with much force. By observing the occlusal activity, we can understand that there is a concentration of energy in the lateral pterygoid muscles sufficient to cause a tissue response there. Remembering this process, we can many times get a good background for understanding not necessarily the microscopic pathologic changes in the tissues themselves, because we can't see them in the clinic, but of the signs and symptoms that we should then try to analyze. Thank you.

*Dr. Solberg*

I would like now to go to the speakers' table for any remarks that they would care to make.

*Dr. Mahan*

Dr. *Moffett,* you were talking about the fact that the first symptoms to appear clinically are those of dysfunction, and that clinical signs of morphologic alterations are not seen until later. I certainly agree that that is the case. I think there is perhaps an exception that is often a problem to the dentist. I refer to cases of degenerative arthritis where advanced changes have occurred and the patient has gone along fat, dumb and happy, with no problems at all until their dentist seats a three unit bridge, and as they bite down on that bite stick to seat that bridge something "snaps" up in the TMJ–now they've got pain. Three months later we see them and they know the three unit bridge is causing their pain. In this instance the patient had morphological changes before they became fully aware of the symptom. However, I certainly agree that the generalization you made is true.

*Dr. Moffett*

Yes, it is rare that you can document only one stimulus–response relationship. They are usually multiple and I think for the patient's benefit and ours, from the medicolegal point of view, we have got to really document and try to get the time perspective identified as to when each of these multiple stimuli might have entered into the picture. It seems to me that the principles that we are talking about must be recognized in dental practice whether or not you intentionally wish to diagnose and deal with TMJ problems. The milieu that we live in today makes it very advisable for a dentist working on the jaws, in any context whatsoever, to establish some kind of biologic baseline before he does something, whether or not he wants to become involved in the subject we are talking about today.

*Dr. Mahan*

Yes, I think if the restorative dentist is going to do a lot of occlusal treatment for a middle-aged female, he ought to take three minutes to diagnose the joint, just listen to it, palpate it but maybe not having to X-ray it, as you point out, as I am against unnecessary X-rays. It just takes three minutes, really, to examine that joint superficially and determine whether there may be morphological changes.

*Dr. Moffett*

I could expand on Dr. *Mahan*'s comment in that not only can one see this degree of degenerative change without the patient having been aware of it, but also individuals who have had inflammatory arthritis, like rheumatoid arthritis, can end up in the TMJ clinic for some problem of jaw function. Then we can often document radiographically that their TMJs show extensive degenerative changes caused by this inflammatory arthritis, even though their jaw joints didn't bother them like the other joints usually do in rheumatoid arthritis. So not only can degenerative breakdown of the TMJ be relatively asymptomatic, but it is frightening how much rheumatoid arthritic changes can occur in the TMJ without a level of symptoms approaching the intensity of pain and discomfort that one sees in other joints affected by rheumatoid. So, for that reason, I think that just the history of rheumatoid arthritis, even if the patient says her jaw joints never bothered her, makes it obligatory to get a good radiograph of such a patient's TMJs.

*Dr. Mahan*

If I may make one more comment concerning Dr. *Krogh-Poulson*'s mentioning of his observations in the Class II. Division 1 and Class II, Division 2 cases. Ingervall studied these cases extensively, and he demonstrated that the slide from retruded contact position to intercuspal position is up and forward in the Class II, Division 1 and 2, just like in all of us normal folks, but that these subjects hold their jaw down and forward in rest position: the Division 2 further down than the usual 3 mm or so, maybe 4 or 5 mm, and the Division 1 more down and forward. So he felt that they are holding their mandibles, at rest, in a forward position for mechanical reasons, or to keep the flies out and that sort of thing, so that their lateral pterygoids are working excessively. When you work muscles like in the jogger, his hamstrings foreshorten. If you function a muscle at a shorter length, those muscles will indeed become spastic and shorten and they are much more liable to injury. I think this goes along with what was said in terms of lateral pterygoid problems.

*Dr. Laskin*

I would like to first compliment Dr. *Moffett* on really a well-organized approach to many of the things that we, as clinicians, have been doing sort of intuitively for a long period of time. However, I think that some of his comments have to be put in proper perspective, because although we are focusing here today on essentially internal derangements of the temporomandibular joint, I don't want the audience to go away thinking that, in terms of incidence, people with grating joints represent the major portion of patients that we see. I am also concerned about the fact that right now we are in a stage where we are making assumptions. We are looking at new types of radiographs, we are getting back into arthrography, and we are looking at autopsy material where we don't really have histories on patients. So I think we are really in a very early stage in our thinking and a lot of this is speculative, at least as far as I am concerned, in terms of its ultimate meaning. Not that we shouldn't be thinking in these directions, but we have to temper our thinking with the established basic concepts. Also, what was not pointed out, or was not emphasized strongly enough, is that the emphasis was on organic problems and a lot of the clicking and popping that we see, I think, represent functional problems. So I would hate to see the emphasis put on repair of the meniscus and procedures of this sort, in areas where we really are dealing with a functional disorder. Finally I would take issue with the statement about the overuse of radiographs. I think it is a truism, that we shouldn't overuse radiographs on patients. On the other hand, I don't think any dentist in this room would rely only on his clinical examination to decide what teeth needed restoration. He would at least take some bite wings to see if there is any incipient caries, and I think a patient with a temporomandibular joint disorder deserves the same type of care. Although the incidence of organic pathology outside of the possibility of degenerative changes in the temporomandibular joint is not great in patients that we see, it would be regretable to perform reconstruction or equilibration on a patient who really has some serious organic change.

*Dr. Moffett*

I think I could probably debate effectively, on the basis of clinical judgment and biologic information, those points of view, and respond to them in different ways. For instance, just because a small percentage of TMJ patients might have the kind of problem that I have been talking about, in no way lessens the need to deal with that problem. I'm not trying to extend it and say that this is **the** problem. I am pointing to ones that are most neglected, and most neglected by individuals in your field, by the way. I am focusing attention on the individuals who need to have a completely different kind of management by people in your field than they are getting at the present time. It doesn't have to be the majority of individuals. I am focusing again on the approach to diagnosis. I am talking about a patient who comes in with a problem even though he may not have the most common problem that comes through the door. He is the most neglected and most poorly understood patient in that total bag of different kinds of problems. You may not choose to focus upon him because he isn't the most common one, but I hope other members in your specialty will, in fact, begin to do so just because he is the most neglected, abused, poorly managed kind of patient. He doesn't have to be the most numerous, in my opinion, to warrant our consideration.

*Dr. Solberg*

We will have to close the discussion from the table and take only one question from the floor. Your name, please.

*Dr. Baers* (Los Angeles, California)

I am *Harry Baers,* an otologist who had my early training under Dr. *James Costen.* I would like to ask Dr. *Moffett* two questions. Among the symptomatology listed, no reference was ever made about any hearing loss or tinnitus, which of course Dr. *Costen* listed in his early description of his syndrome. I would like to ask Dr. *Moffett* about a recent anatomical work that has shown by special electron microscopy and special staining, sympathetic innervation of the cochlea which for years was denied. A reflex arc was revealed with sympathetic nerve fibers that could be originating in the TMJ and eventually ending up in the cochlea and could give us an anatomical explanation for tinnitus. Have you had any information or documentation or listing about these two syndromes?

*Dr. Moffett*

No, I haven't. I commend you on looking in these directions, because this is another part of the potential progress that lies ahead of us. I think the opportunity for the clinician to see how these problems might be handled in a mutually beneficial way, for the jaw joint and the hearing and equilibrium mechanisms directly adjacent to it, offers more promise for the future than can be realized right now with our existing explanations. A good clinician can collect information on responses to clinical treatment that will tell us what we had better investigate further in the laboratory. It makes perfect sense for you to seek out the possibilities of dealing with these mutually inter-related problems, and then, hopefully, the nonclinicians will get the message and will begin to concentrate more on trying to explain it. If you continue thinking along these lines and recording and documenting responses, that will compel us to take a look in this area, and I think we should.

# II. The Temporomandibular Joint in Function and Pathofunction

by Parker E. Mahan

In order to discuss the function and pathofunction of the temporomandibular joint (TMJ), one must first describe the many details of its anatomy. No joint could demonstrate the correlation of structure and function more precisely than does the TMJ. This freely movable joint contains two cavities whose articular surfaces are not hyaline cartilage as seen in most joints of the body. The articular surfaces of the mandibular fossa, articular eminence and condyle are comprised essentially of collagen (see Fig. 1). There are small areas of cartilage cells seen on the crest of the articular eminence, but on the condyle the secondary cartilage is completely covered by collagen. The central portion of the meniscus is also comprised of collagen fibers, organized in sheets of anterior-posteriorly oriented fibers on the superior and inferior surfaces, and oriented in all three directions in space[24] in the central areas (Fig. 2). Chondroid cells have been identified in menisci from subjects over 30 years of age but there are no parallel rows of chondrocytes in a cartilagenous matrix as seen in hyaline cartilage[19]. The pliable meniscus is thus able to support stabilization of the condyle against the articular eminence even though the embrasure between the two bones varies greatly as the condyle translates from a concave fossa to a convex eminence. This function could not be served by a stiff, cartilagenous meniscus. The synovial tissues that line the periphery of the superior cavity appear as villi in sagittal sections of the joint. The posterior villi are actually folds of synovial membrane that are attached along the squamotympanic suture in the temporal bone and to the superior surface of the pars posterior of the meniscus[11,14]. These folds allow the meniscus to translate as far as 2 cm anteriorly by unfolding into a sheet with translation of the condyle. The synovial tissues of the inferior cavity are also folded into villi, allowing the meniscus to rotate posteriorly as the condyle translates forward. Lymphatic capillaries, located in the synovial villi, provide serum for the creation of the small amount of synovial fluid necessary to lubricate the articular surfaces of the joint. When one inserts a needle into the superior and inferior cavities of the healthy TMJ, synovial fluid cannot be aspirated. However, the passive fill volume of the superior cavity averages 1.2 ml and that of the inferior cavity averages 0.9 ml[27]. It has been shown in 11 patients with hypermobility of the TMJ that there is a 60 % increase in the superior cavity passive fill volume (1.9 ml) and a 20 % increase in the inferior cavity (1.1 ml)[27].

The posterior attachments of the meniscus, which are very complicated, are part of the region known as the bilaminar zone because it contains two strata of fibers with loose, areolar connective tissue filling the space between them (Fig. 2). The superior stratum is attached to the tympanic plate and is com-

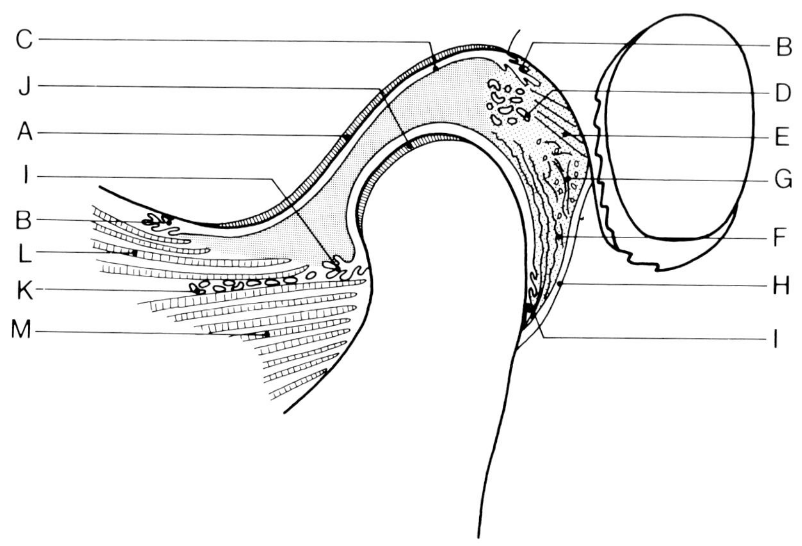


Fig. 1 Sagittal view of the TMJ.

A-Articular surface of the temporal bone, B-Synovial membrane of superior cavity, C-Superior cavity, D-Vascular knee, E-Superior stratum of bilaminar zone, F-Inferior stratum of bilaminar zone, G-Loose areolar connective tissue, H-Posterior capsule, I-Inferior cavity synovial membrane, J-Articular surface of condyle, K-Blood vessels, L-Superior belly of lateral pterygoid, M-Inferior belly of lateral pterygoid muscle.

prised of elastin rather than collagen[10]. Elastin is the only fibrous protein of the body that has a true modulus of elasticity. Since, in the healthy TMJ, the meniscus is tightly attached to the medial and lateral pole of the condyle[7], its attachment to bone posteriorly must be elastic to allow the meniscus to translate forward with the condyle. When the TMJ has been freed by incising the two bellies of the lateral pterygoid and sectioning the neck of the condylar process in a cadaver, the action of the superior stratum of the bilaminar zone can be easily demonstrated. If one grasps the neck of the condylar process, displaces the condyle down onto the eminence and then releases his grasp, the condyle will rapidly snap back into the fossa. The inferior stratum of the bilaminar zone is not stretched as the condyle translates forward because the meniscus rotates posteriorly, relieving any tension in this stratum. Above the postero-superior aspect of the condyle, and anterior to the bilaminar zone, the meniscus is very vascular. This region, called the vascular knee (genu vasculosa)[10], may contain glomus cell arteriovenous shunts. Actually, blood vessels completely encircle the avascular central area of the meniscus, with blood being shunted back and forth with jaw function to compensate for the volume of the condyle as it vacates one space and fills another[1,5]. The anterior extension of the

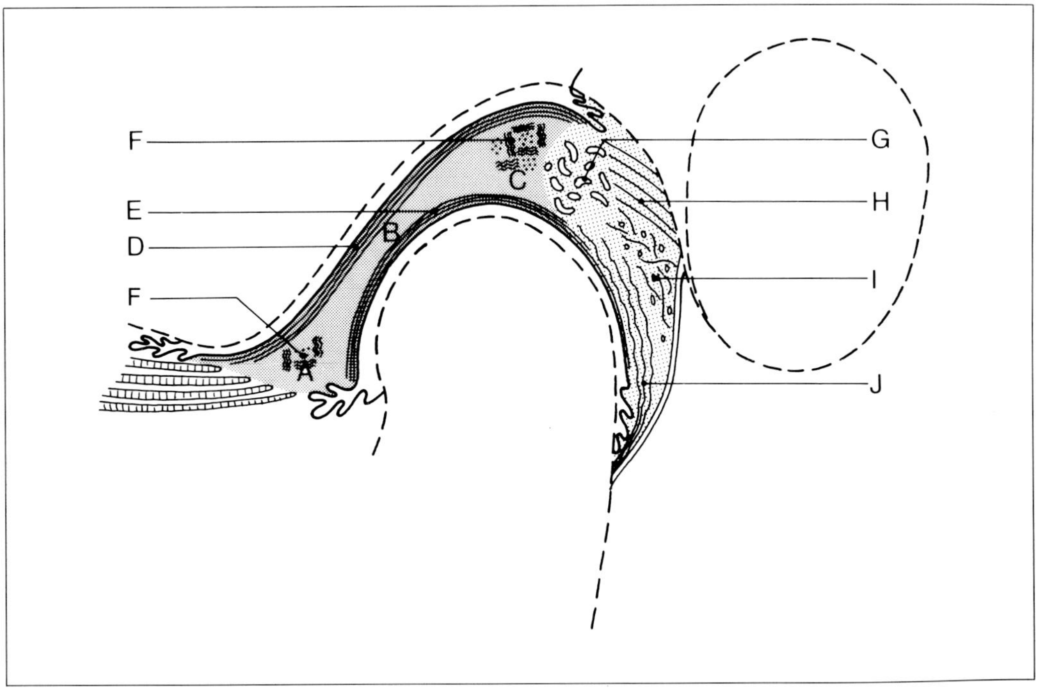


Fig. 2 Details of TMJ meniscus anatomy.

A-Foot of meniscus (Pes), B-Thin, avascular part (Pars Gracilis), C-Pars posterior, D-Sheet of parallel collagen fibers on superior surface, E-Sheet of parallel collagen fibers on inferior surface, F-Zones of collagen fibers oriented in all three directions, G-Vascular knee, H-Superior stratum of bilaminar zone, I-Loose areolar connective tissue, vessels and nerves, J-Inferior stratum of bilaminar zone.

mensicus at its attachment to the superior belly of the lateral pterygoid is also very vascular. These blood vessels supply the two bellies of the lateral pterygoid muscle as well as the joint structures. At the time of birth the entire meniscus and the superior surface of the condyle are vascularized[4], with the central region of the meniscus becoming avascular by age three to five. The fetal condyle is penetrated by vascular canals with blood vessels which anastomose over the articular surface, and then normally disappear by age three.

There is no capsule at the medial half of the anterior aspect of the TMJ and thus, the synovial membrane lining the superior cavity anterior wall is supported only by loose areolar connective tissue. The tissue that forms a capsule-like structure at the lateral half of the anterior aspect of the joint is not well organized into a thick sheet of collagen fibers but is also loose areolar connective tissue. This lack of an anterior capsule comprises the anatomical "Achilles heel" of the TMJ. Hypertranslation of the condyle cannot be prevented by a sturdy anterior capsule, so, trauma to the synovial tissues and lateral pterygoid muscle attachments occurs. This anatomical feature is probably responsible for the high incidence of TMJ pain and dysfunction following whiplash injury. With rapid extension of the head in a whiplash, the

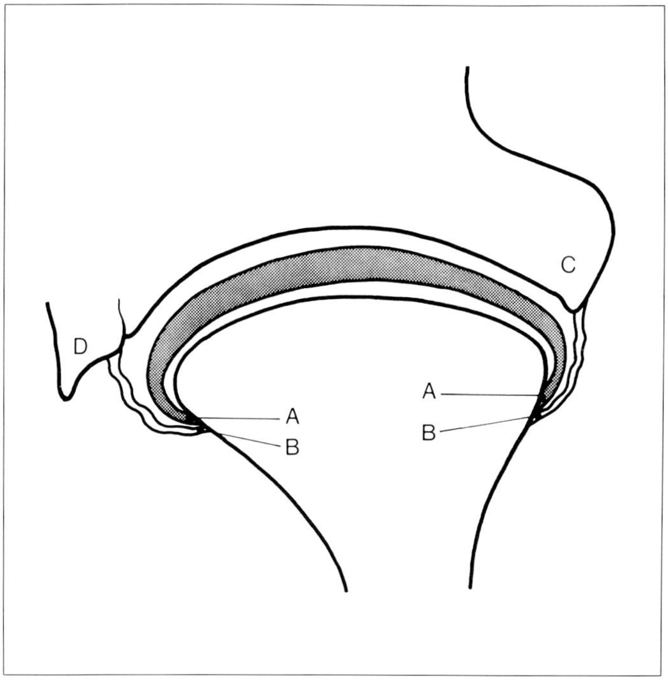


Fig. 3 Frontal view of TMJ indicating attachments of the meniscus and capsules: A-Tight attachment of meniscus to medial and lateral pole of the condyle, B-Attachment of capsule to medial and lateral poles of condyle, C-Lateral lip of glenoid fossa, D-Spinous process of sphenoid bone.

supra and infrahyoid muscles cannot lengthen rapidly enough so they hold back on the mandibular symphysis whipping the condyles forward excessively. The posterior deep temporal nerves, located on the temporal bone just anterior to the articular eminence, lie in the path of hypertranslation of the condyles and could thus be traumatized.

The capsule on the medial and lateral wall of the joint is comprised of collagen but the fibers are not under tension (Fig. 3). This laxity in the fiber arrangements does not firmly support the joint but allows the medial and lateral poles of the condyles to translate forward without tearing the capsule.

Unlike the capsular attachments, the meniscus is tightly attached to the lateral and medial poles of the condyle in the healthy TMJ. There will be no meniscus-condyle discoordination with joint clicking or popping unless these attachments are loosened or torn.

If one dissects the superior cavity of a healthy TMJ at its periphery, leaving the meniscus attached to the condyle, one can gain a clear understanding of the function between these structures. By holding the neck of the condylar process and placing a sharp probe into the exposed, superior surface of the meniscus, one can demonstrate little or no lateral movement of the meniscus but complete rotation anterior and posterior to the condyle.

When the capsule is excised over the lateral pole of the condyle, one gains access to the superior cavity of the joint. The meniscus must then be released from its tight attachment at the lateral pole in order to enter the inferior cavity. It follows that the meniscus should not be sutured to the capsule in closing TMJ surgery, since this attachment would fix the lateral aspect of the mensicus to the lateral lip of the glenoid fossa. When such a post surgical patient attempted to open widely and translate the condyle, the meniscus would be normally bound to the medial pole but not at the lateral pole. Attempted condylar translation would then tense the meniscus from the condylar medial pole to the lateral lip of the glenoid fossa thus limiting translation and deflecting the meniscus off the lateral pole as it moved forward. The capsule of the TMJ is well organized on the posterior wall, and extends from the tympanic plate to the neck of the condylar process.

A number of structures actually pass through the TMJ. In the medial aspect of the glenoid fossa where the squamotympanic, petrotympanic and squamopetrosal sutures meet, the anterior tympanic artery, chorda tympani nerve and a fibroelastic ligament enter the superior cavity. The ligament, the anterior malleolar ligament, is attached to the anterior process of the malleus superiorly and blends into the capsule and sphenomandibular ligament inferiorly[6]. TMJ surgery has been associated with a tearing of the posterior-superior quadrant of the tympanic membrane and a reduction of hearing by 80 %. This trauma results from tension on the anterior malleolar ligament via the sphenomandibular ligament as the mandible is depressed inferiorly by instrumentation.

The collateral ligament of the joint, called the temporomandibular ligament, extends from the lateral and inferior surface of the zygomatic arch to the lateral neck of the condylar process. The posterior and inferior direction of this ligament allows it to function like a pendulum during translation of the condyle so that it will resist excessive lateral condylar displacement and still allow forward translation. A deep, horizontal band of the temporomandibular ligament may extend from the crest of the articular tubercle to the lateral pole of the condyle[23].

The medial, posterior and lateral walls of the TMJ capsule and the lateral half of the anterior wall are innervated by a large branch of the auriculotemporal nerve as it crosses posterior to the neck of the condylar process[25]. Blocking this nerve just posterior to the condylar neck will usually anaesthetize the TMJ. The posterior deep temporal and masseteric nerves supply the anterior region of the joint but most of their fibers are larger than the C and A delta fibers that subserve pain.

Studies in both monkey and man have demonstrated that the two bellies of the lateral pterygoid muscle function as antagonistic muscles[18, 16]. The large inferior belly contracts on mouth opening and the superior belly contracts on closing. The inferior belly extends from the pterygoid fovea in the neck of the condylar process, inferiorly and medially to the lateral surface of the lateral pterygoid plate. When it contracts, it translates the condyle down onto the articular eminence and pulls medially. The superior belly attaches to the anterior margin of the meniscus and to the deep fibers of the inferior belly posteriorly. It takes origin from the floor of the infratemporal fossa. It is also directed medially and serves to pull the meniscus anteriorly and medially. Since the superior belly does not contract on mouth opening, the tight attachment of the meniscus to the medial and lateral poles of the condyle are the only factors that maintain a functional relation between the meniscus and condyle during condylar translation. As the condyle translates anteriorly in a healthy joint, the elastic superior stratum of the bilaminar zone will hold back on the meniscus tending to rotate it posteriorly and applying tension on its attachments at the condy-

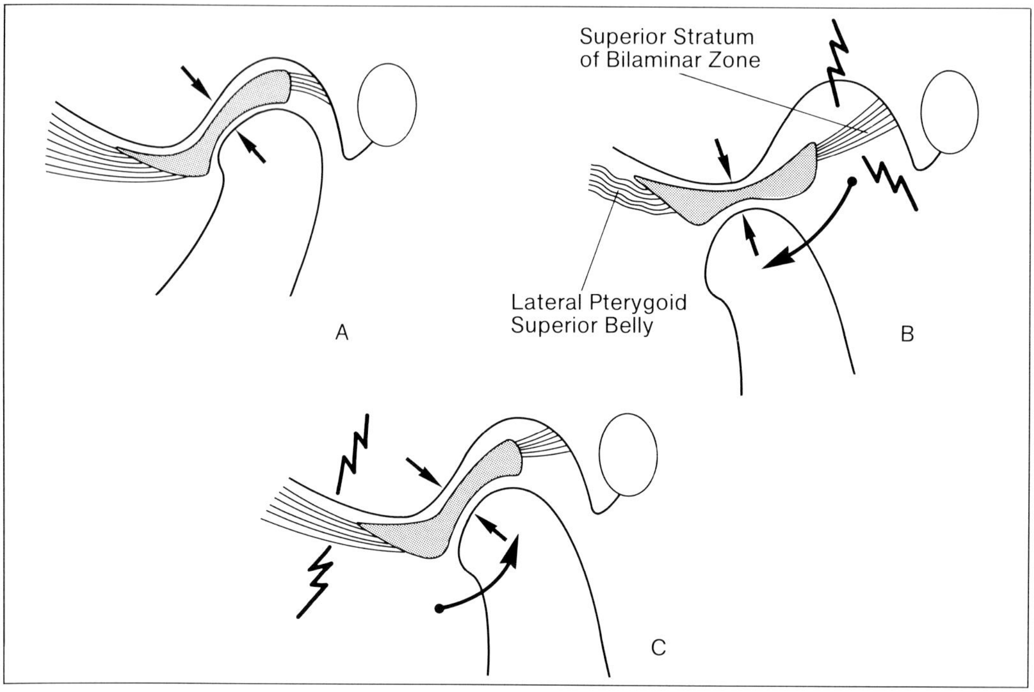


Fig. 4 Drawing of meniscus position during rest (A), opening movement (B), and closing movement (C). Note that during mouth opening, (B), as the condyle translates anteriorly onto the eminence, the superior belly of the lateral pterygoid is not contracting and tension in the superior stratum of the bilaminar zone has rotated the meniscus posteriorly on the condyle. The small arrows indicate location of maximum pressure on the articular surfaces. During closure of the mouth, (C), as the condyle translates posteriorly, the superior belly of the lateral pterygoid is active, holding anteriorly on the meniscus and placing it back onto the antero-superior surface of the condyle while counteracting the pull of the superior stratum.

lar poles. If the bilaminar zone has been destroyed or degenerated as a result of trauma or joint disease and if the tight attachments at the condylar poles are loosened or torn, the tonus of the superior belly could displace the meniscus anteriorly. This would produce an increased joint space anterior to the condyle in lateral TMJ radiographs and laminagraphs, and would also result in an anterior radio-opaque zone in inferior cavity arthrograms during wide opening of the mouth. This subject will be discussed at length in two other papers of this symposium.

It seems that the posterior rotation of the mensicus during condylar translation as a result of superior stratum elastic tension will keep the thin part of the meniscus between the condyle and articular eminence where maximum pressure is exerted (Fig. 4). However, during closure of the mouth, the elastic tension is still in effect and the meniscus would tend to be pushed back up into the posterior region of the fossa unless the superior belly of the lateral pterygoid began contracting to hold forward on the meniscus during mouth closure. Thus, we have the interaction of a passive tension-producing

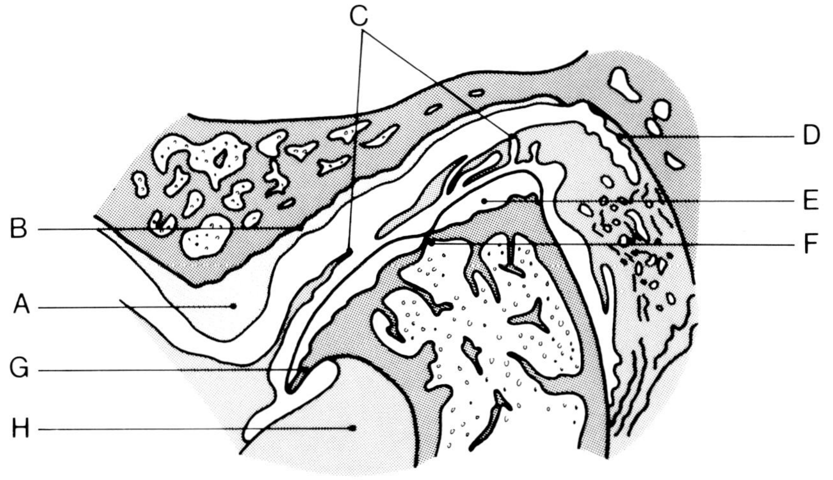


Fig. 5 Drawing of TMJ with degenerative arthritis (TMJ arthrosis) A-Build up of collagen over articular eminence, B-Flattened and eroded articular eminence, C-Remnants of meniscus, D-Synovial membrane, E-Collagenous surface of condyle, F-Degenerated articular surface of condyle, G-Osteophyte, H-Fibers of lateral pterygoid inferior belly.

tissue (superior stratum of the bilaminar zone) and an active tension-producing tissue (superior belly of the lateral pterygoid) acting upon the meniscus to keep it functionally related to the condyle during mouth opening and closing. This interaction will usually fail, however, if the tight attachment of the meniscus to the condylar poles has been loosened or torn. Clicking and popping joint sounds are usually associated with meniscus-condyle discoordination[27, 28, 8], and is usually easily detected by palpation just anterior to the tragus of the ear during mouth opening and lateral deviation of the mandible.

Degenerative arthritis of the TMJ usually affects one side at a time and is signaled by pain on movement of the condyle. Indeed, many of these patients will open 20 mm in the centric relation arc but will not open further because condylar translation is painful. In most cases, this pain goes away in 8 months[26, 14, 15]. Joint changes in this disease include flattening of the condyle and articular eminence, narrowing of the joint space, dystrophic calcification or lipping at the periphery of the degenerated articular surfaces, formation of Ely's cysts in the degenerated articular surfaces, zones of

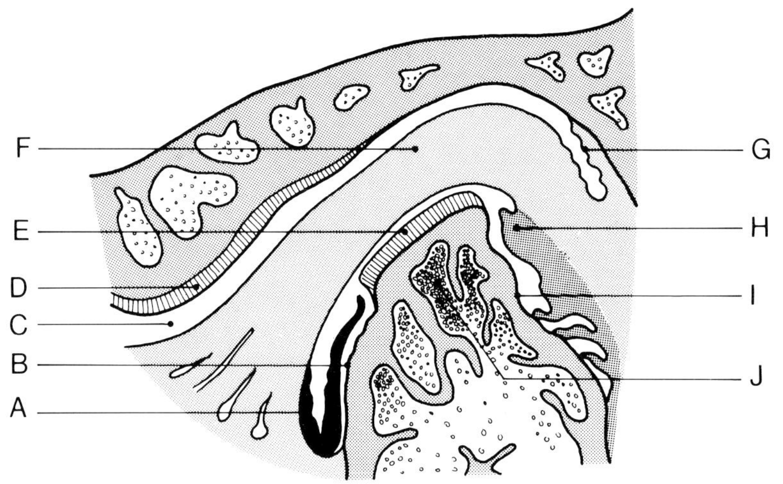


Fig. 6 Drawing of TMJ with rheumatoid arthritis. A-Pannus eroding condyle from the anterior, B-Eroded condylar bone, C-Superior cavity, D-Collagenous articular surface of articular eminence, E-Remaining, normal articular collagen on condyle, F-Unaffected (normal) collagen of the meniscus, G-Synovial membrane of superior cavity (not yet affected by pannus formation), H-Newly formed collagen from pannus, I-Eroded bone on posterior of condyle, J-Acute inflammation.

sclerotic bone at the surfaces, fibrillation and perforation of the meniscus and a coarse or fine crepitus upon condylar translation (Fig. 5). These changes usually occur over a one to three year period and then the joint returns to almost normal, painless function with continued crepitus. It is amazing how little occlusal adjustment is required following these joint changes in most patients. A smaller, unlucky group remain troubled by painful TMJ function and must seek relief in surgery or chronic medication.

The actual etiology of degenerative arthritis is still unknown but some interesting studies have shown that impact loading of joints, rather than sliding and gliding movements, will result in changes that mimic those of degenerative arthritis[22]. When the hind legs of rabbits are placed in acrylic splints and an eccentric wheel displaces the leg superiorly into the acetabulum once a second for an hour a day, the hip joints show changes like degenerative arthritis within 30 days. These changes include lipping of the articular surface, fibrillation and breaking up of the articular cartilage, and loss of acid mucopolysaccharide staining in the cartilage.

When a patient loses posterior teeth up to the first premolars without their replacement, mastication or clenching will tend to impact load the TMJ's. On closure in such a patient, a fulcrum is produced at the

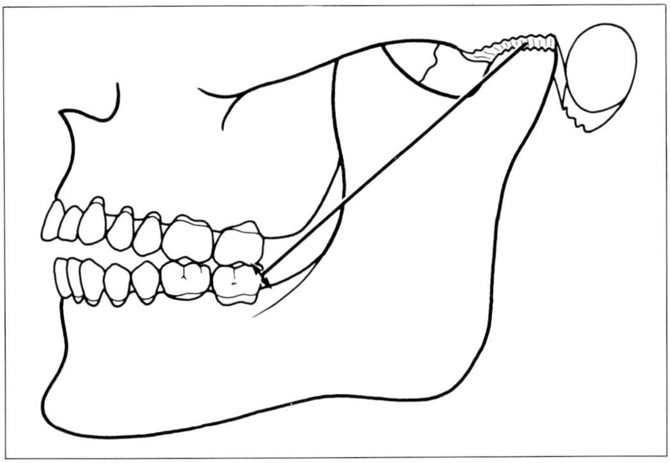

Fig. 7 Drawing of mandibular position resulting from condylar erosion in rheumatoid arthritis. Note fibrous ankylosis and shortened condyle. Closure on the decreased radius results in occlusal contact on the distal of the second molars producing a retruded anterior open bite.

premolars, the mandibular elevator muscles collectively act posteriorly to this fulcrum and the load of the lever arm is exerted between the condyle and the fossa-articular eminence. Such force, driving the bones toward each other, may be related to degenerative changes in the TMJ.

Rheumatoid arthritis on the other hand, tends to affect both TMJ's simultaneously[3]. This disease typically begins at the periphery of the joint as the synovial tissues are converted into pannus cells. These cells release enzymes which erode the condyle and temporal bone from the periphery inward toward the center of the articular surfaces (Fig. 6). Degenerative arthritis progresses in the opposite manner, showing degeneration in the center of the articular surfaces working outward toward the joint periphery. In rheumatoid arthritis, acute inflammation is seen in the marrow spaces beneath the eroding bone. As the pannus cells destroy bone, they are converted to fibroblasts and tend to produce fibrous ankylosis of the joint. As the condyle erodes away, the remaining condylar process moves up into the fossa and becomes ankylosed. This shortens the radius of the mandibular rami so the last pair of molars contact on mouth closure creating an anterior open bite (Fig. 7). With fibrous ankylosis of the TMJ, the maximum mouth opening may approach zero.

Congenital abnormalities may also produce TMJ pathofunction. Bifid condyles have been found to produce painful clicking and joint dysfunction[12]. These abnormalities may result from the separation of the lateral and medial aspects of the developing condyle by the vascular canals and their connective tissue septa that form in the human condyle[20].

Studies in growing monkeys have demonstrated that retrusive elastic forces applied to the mandible will alter the morphology of the TMJ[13, 21], although, the clinical significance of these studies has not yet been determined. Induced malocclusion in monkeys will also affect the morphology of the neck and head of the condylar process[9,2].

Cinefluorographic studies of the human temporomandibular joint have demonstrated that 70 % of the subjects moved their condyles anterior to the articular eminence during wide opening of the mouth[17]. These subjects did not experience subluxation and locking but only had hypermobility. Actually, the articular surface of the eminence extends anterior to its crest and so it may be normal (or usual) to observe such anterior translation of the condyle during maximum opening of the mouth.

## References


1. *Batson, O. B.*
The Anatomist Looks at the Temporomandibular Joint. Trans. Acad. Ophthalmol. Otolaryngol. **60**: 413, 1956.
2. *Baume, L. J.* and *H. Derichsweiler*
Is the Condylar Growth Center Responsive to Orthodontic Therapy? An Experimental Study in Macaca Mulatta. O. Surg., O. Med. O. Path. **14**: 347, 1961.
3. *Blackwood, H. J. J.*
Arthritis of the Mandibular Joint. Brit. Dent. J. **115**: 317, 1963.
4. *Blackwood, H. J. J.*
Vascularization of the Condylar Cartilage of the Human Mandible. J. Anat. **99**: 551, 1965.
5. *Boyer, C. C.,* et al.
Blood Supply of the Temporomandibular Joint. J. Dent. Res. **43**: 224, 1944.
6. *Burch, J. G.*
The Cranial Attachment of the Sphenomandibular (tympanomandibular) Ligament. Anat. Rec. **156**: 433, 1966.
7. *Choukas, N. C.* and *H. Sicher*
The Structure of the Temporomandibular Joint. Oral Surg. **13**: 1203, 1960.
8. *Farrar, W. B.*
Characteristics of the Condylar Path in Internal Derangements of the TMJ. J. Pros. Dent. **39**: 319, 1978.
9. *Gianelly, A. A.* et al
Effect of Experimentally Altered Occusal Vertical Dimension on Temporomandibular Articulation. J. Pros. Dent. **24**: 629, 1970.
10. *Griffin, C. J.* and *C. J. Sharpe*
The Structure of the Adult Human Temporomandibular Meniscus. Aust. Dent. J. **5**: 190, 1960.
11. *Griffin, C. J.* and *C. J. Sharpe*
The Distribution of the Synovial Membrane and Mechanism of its Blood Supply in the Adult Human Temporomandibular Joint. Aust. Dent. J. **5**: 367, 1960.
12. *Grossman, E.*
An Unusual Case of Clicking Jaw. Brit. J. Oral Surg. **3**: 158, 1966.
13. *Janzen, E. K.* and *J. A. Bluher*
The Cephalometric, Anatomic and Histologic Changes in Macaca Mulatta After Application of a Continuous-acting Retraction Force on the Mandible. Am J. Ortho. **51**: 823, 1965.
14. *Kreutziger, K. L.* and *P. E. Mahan*
Temporomandibular Degenerative Joint Disease Part I. Anatomy, Pathophysiology and Clinical Description. O. Surg., O. Med., O. Path. **40**: 165, 1975.
15. *Kreutziger, K. L.* and *P. E. Mahan*
Temporomandibular Degenerative Joint Disease Part II. Diagnostic Procedure and Comprehensive Management. O. Surg., O. Med., O. Path. **40**: 297, 1975
16. *Lipke, D. P.,* et al.
An Electromyographic Study of the Human Lateral Pterygoid Muscle. J. Dent. Res. 56 Special Issue B: B230, 1977 (Abstract No. 713).
17. *McLeran, J. H.,* et al.
A Cinefluorographic Analysis of the Temporomandibular Joint. J. Am Dent. Assoc. **75**: 1394, 1967.
18. *McNamara, J. A.*
The Independent Functions of the Two Heads of the Lateral Pterygoid Muscle. Am J. Anat. **138**: 197, 1973.
19. *Mathews, M. P.* and *B. C. Moffett*
Histologic Maturation and Initial Aging of the Human Temporomandibular Joint. J. Dent. Res. 53 Special Issue: 246, 1974 (Abstract No. 765).
20. *Moffett, B.*
The Morphogenesis of the Temporomandibular Joint. Am. J. Ortho. **52**: 401, 1966.
21. *Payne, G. S.*
The Effect of Intermaxillary Elastic Force on the Temporomandibular Articulation in the Growing Macaque Monkey. Am. J. Ortho. **60**: 491, 1971.
22. *Radin, E. L.,* et al.
Response of Joints to Impact Loading III. Relationships Between Trabecular Microfractures and Cartilage Degeneration. J. Biomechanics **6**: 51, 1973.
23. *Sicher, H.* and *E. L. DuBrul*
Oral Anatomy; Sixth Edition, C. V. Mosby Co. St. Louis. 1975, pp. 164.
24. *Strauss, F.,* et al.
The Architecture of the Disk of the Human Temporomandibular Joint. Helv. Odont. Acta. **4**: 1, 1960.
25. *Thilander, B.*
Innervation of the Temporomandibular Joint Capsule in Man. Trans. Roy, Schools Stoch. Umea No **7**: 1, 1961.
26. *Toller, P. A.*
Osteoarthrosis of the Mandibular Condyle. Brit. Dent. J. **134**: 223, 1973.
27. *Toller, P. A.*
Opaque Arthrography of the Temporomandibular Joint. Int. J. Oral Surg. **3**: 17, 1974.
28. *Yavelow, I.* and *G. S. Arnold*
Temporomandibular Joint Clicking. Oral Surg. **32**: 708, 1971.

# Discussion

Discussant: Torsten Öberg

*Dr. Öberg*

Thank you for a very fine lecture; I've learned much in this hour. I am glad to hear that you believe the attachment of the disc to the condyle allows rotation in a sagittal direction with relatively little side play. In our autopsy material, we have also found the disc very firm in its attachment. The literature, for example *Rees* (1954), implies that there is a rather wide range of relative movement between the condyle and the disc, but I think this arrangement exists only when you have a pathological condition.
I also agree that the bellies of the lateral pterygoid muscle can function independently of each other. This is very important for understanding the nature of some forms of locking and clicking.
But I also want to ask you a question. If there is loss of molar support with a consequent backward positioning of the condyle, is it possible that the condyle might function behind the posterior dense part of the disc? What do you think of this hypothetical sequence of events and its relationship to clicking?

*Dr. Mahan*

Dr. *Öberg* and I decided that we would tell it like it is and then we could straighten out each other's interpretations; that is what we are doing here. I agree with your description and in cases where we have lack of posterior support, like when the second premolars are the last centric stops, a fulcrum is produced at those pairs of contacts. The usual position and direction of the elevator muscles (masseter, medial pterygoid and temporalis) is about the region of the mesiobuccal cusp of the first molar in an upward and slightly forward direction. That means we are producing a lever with a fulcrum anterior to the force. So now the force is elevated and the load is then applied against the posterior incline of the articular eminence and, as you point out, driving the condyle and disc components up and backward into the mandibular fossa. I think the loss of posterior support could constitute a pattern of dysfunction in which excessive stresses applied against the meniscus could cause degeneration of its central part. It is also possible to get pathological changes in what I call the vascular knee, or the bilaminar zone, and bring about degeneration in that region. So I agree with you, and this draws us into some philosophical questions as well. Should we put partial dentures in a patient's mouth and give him posterior teeth with the risk that he is going to tear up his abutment teeth? That is a professional decision that we have to make today in our practice.

*Dr. Öberg*

There may be other causes of clicking in addition to muscular incoordination and condyle-disc displacement. We have found that there can be a clinically significant deviation in form of the condyle (remodeling), with secondary cupping-out of localized areas on the disc. Under rotation and translation of the condyle against the disc, the clicking sound could be produced. In my opinion, remodeling can be a third cause of clicking. The devation in form due to remodeling is also the result of an altered biomechanical loading in the joint and perhaps we could speak more about that later . . .

I would like to comment on other things. You have told us that there is no cartilage in the disc after 20–30 years.

*Dr. Mahan*

Dr. *Moffett* shows chondroid cells in dystrophic cartilage.

*Dr. Öberg*

It is important to know that there exist cartilage cells because they are producing aggregates of proteoglycans which are responsible for the ability of the disc to resist pressure and wear and tear.

*Dr. Mahan*

To make it brittle? . . . is that what you mean?

*Dr. Öberg*

No, proteoglycans are very important for the elasticity of the disc.

*Dr. Mahan*

Being a nonhistologist and not being bothered by the facts, I call that hyalinization of collagen. Dr. *Moffett* will comment on this.

*Dr. Öberg*

Well, hyalinization is another thing for me. I think that hyalinization implies the presence of real chrondroid cells.

*Dr. Moffett*

In this change I don't think one sees the same loss of integrity of the collagen bundles as when we compress the periodontal joints and get hyalinization or a type of aseptic necrosis. I do think that collagen bundles in the disc are still intact and it is just a phenomenon in which the cells there take on the histologic appearance of cartilage cells in a fibrous matrix if indeed they are not chondrocytes. So I think there is a difference in the way we use the term hyalinization, in orthodontics to mean a breakdown or loss of the histologic structure of the collagen fibers. Hyalinization might occur under some instances but it usually doesn't seem to be associated with the development of these cartilage cells.

*Dr. Solberg*

I think we need further clarification. Are you both saying there is no translation or sliding of the condyle against the inferior portion of the meniscus? I want that clarified one way or the other.

*Dr. Mahan*

My feeling is that rotation occurs in the healthy joint. That is, any given point on the condyle is indeed moving relative to the inferior aspect of the meniscus. But I am also calling it rotation as the meniscus moves forward so there isn't nearly the extent of shearing occurring between the two surfaces in the inferior cavity as there is in the superior cavity. We break it down into translation and rotation, but even the rotation means that the articular surface of the condyle is rubbing against the inferior aspect of the meniscus in an anterior direction on opening and posterior direction on closing. There is a parallel sheet of collagen fibers on the inferior aspect of the disc just as there is on the superior aspect. That was my feeling.

*Dr. Öberg*

I agree with you.

*Dr. Solberg*

Is the lateral pterygoid muscle part of the temporomandibular joint?

*Dr. Mahan*

It could be semantics, I guess, but I would like to go ahead and say yes. Its tendon is an integral part of the meniscus and you can consider its tendon being in the joint.

*Dr. Laskin*

Just one comment Dr. *Mahan,* and that concerns the work of *S. L. Block* (IADR Abstracts, 1976) on barohypoacusis which gives you another possible explanation for some of the symptoms that patients who have dysfunction of the masticatory apparatus may experience. What *Block* postulated, and his study supported, was the fact that normally there is a relationship between the medial pterygoid muscle and the eustachian tube where the muscle rests against the tube and keeps it in a closed position. The muscle has to be in a relaxed state in order for the eustachian tube to be actively opened, and should spasm, swelling, or edema in the medial pterygoid muscle develop, the eustachian tube will remain closed. This could give rise to some of the stuffiness and other symptoms that TMJ patients have in their ears.

*Dr. Glenn Clark*

Dr. *Mahan,* do you think that orthodontic patients have a higher instance of intracapsular temporomandibular joint problems than a normal population?

*Dr. Mahan*

Dr. *Krogh-Poulsen's* data indicates that among pain patients you see a higher percentage of Class II division 1 and Class II division 2 than you see in the general population.

*Dr. Clark*

How about postorthodontic treatment patients?

*Dr. Mahan*

I don't know if there is data that would indicate that we see more postorthodontic patients. In Umeå Sweden, a very good statistical study with 1100 subjects was performed. It was determined that 39 per cent of the people have clicking and popping. A lot of those people probably were postorthodontic patients. In any event there is a lot of clicking and popping when you learn that two out of five people seated in your chair have joint sounds.

*Dr. Glenn Clark*

I wanted to ask Dr. *Moffett* if he would comment on the incidence of intracapsular problems in postorthodontic treatment patients. In other words, if a patient has a malocclusion, is he running a higher risk of developing symptoms by having a treatment than remaining untreated?

*Dr. Moffett*

No, I don't think that is the case. I think that if you believe in occlusal biology you ought to apply it, whether the TMJ's are involved or not. It doesn't make sense to me to say, "well, I am not going to correct this problem because I may be creating more of a problem then I did before I started." In dentistry, I think you have to decide what you believe and practice it. That goes, not only for orthodontics, but for restorative dentistry or any other area. Now, having said that, I think any time we perform any dental treatment for a patient involving physical manipulation of the jaw, the patient is at risk and the joint is at risk. I don't care how careful you are. Unless you do something to reduce the risk before dental treatment begins, you are going to have problems. I guess you can just start applying principles of musculoskeletal conditioning to this part of the musculoskeletal system as we do to the rest of it. The patient would benefit and you would be introducing a preventive concept in dental treatment which isn't in the state of the art at the present time.

Added to the physical risk of mechanical injury involved in restorative dentistry is the fact that when you are changing jaw function you are creating a degree of instability during the process of changing the jaw relationships. The joint is not designed anatomically in a way that it maintains a stable articulation in these instances, especially when the occlusion is being changed dramatically by orthodontic techniques. You are introducing a risk that is purely aside from the question of mechanical forces. The orthodontic patient is going through a biologically unstable period, but to some extent this is equally true for any treatment that changes occlusal biology, and I think you have to weigh that.

You can't stop in the middle. You have to try to monitor these things during treatment to see if you are making a problem worse; if so, you can back off temporarily. What can you do to ease the stress that you are imposing by dental treatment? What can you do to prevent these problems from happening? Can you increase the biological responses in this joint and muscles by some kind of conditioning procedure? All of us ought to be considering these questions just as we do now for the rest of the muscular system.

*Dr. Donald Jones* (New Jersey)

Dr. *Mahan,* would you clarify the function of the superior belly of the lateral pterygoid?

*Dr. Mahan*

I would be happy to, because I went quickly past that. When the patient opens his mouth, elastic tension builds up from the superior stratum of the bilaminar zone holding back the meniscus. Now, if that passive tension is unopposed during the closing motion the disc would be pulled in back of the condyle and up into the fossa. That needs to be counteracted. So what happens is that the superior belly of the lateral pterygoid contracts to maintain the relation of the disc to the condyle as the condyle resumes it position in the fossa. So, the action of the passive tension (posterior) and the active tension (anterior) acts beautifully to keep the meniscus where most of the stress is centered, between the condyle and the temporal bone.

In summary, my idea is that the superior belly of the lateral pterygoid actually directs the meniscus back into position as the condyle translates back into the fossa on closure, counteracting the everpresent passive retrusive force of the elastic superior stratum of the bilaminar zone.

*Dr. William Scheerer* (Honolulu, Hawaii)

A question regarding the passage of the long buccal nerve through the lateral pterygoid. How can you be sure that the pressure from the muscles is causing the paresthesia? Secondly, how do you treat it?

*Dr. Mahan*

I didn't mean to say that we know that that occurs. I said that the long buccal nerve comes out between the two bellies of the lateral pterygoid and if we have disruption in the joint we can actively involve the two bellies of the lateral pterygoid. Now you are getting into the region where you are mechanically interfering with that nerve. A number of patients have told me that they have this weird tingling around the cheek and that is my hypothesis in explaining this. The way we try to treat it depends upon the etiology. Which of the situations do we have? Do we have the hypermobility problem or just a hyperirritability of the lateral pterygoid muscles? We would treat an occlusal problem or the intraarticular problem if there were degenerative changes, or it could be a surgical approach, depending upon the case. If we had, for example, anterior displacement of the meniscus as Dr. *McCarty* will demonstrate, we would treat that with a surgical procedure. In another case where we are just dealing with a hypertrophied superior and inferior belly due to abnormal functioning of the two, then we would go to the treatment that would alleviate that type of hyperfunction. That might be an occlusal splint, occlusal adjustment, reconstruction, or whatever. We said diagnosis depends upon the specific case and this is the case in point.

*Dr. Krogh-Poulsen*

My comment concerns cases where we have a click. In the dissection materials I have been able to demonstrate clicking. When we move the condyle forward and backwards and don't put any upward pressure on it, it won't click. If we apply an upward pressure the disc may get stuck. If you move the condyle a little more forward, you will have a sudden acceleration of the disc causing a click. This would suggest, but this is just a suggestion, that in patients who have clicking you have an extensive activity of the elevators going on all the time. Examples of this are the patients who brux in a forward or lateral position and therefore have a habitual hyperactivity of the elevators. What do you think about that, Dr. *Mahan?*

*Dr. Mahan*

I think that is entirely consistent with our observations and with that of *Paul Toller*'s, in that it appears that the meniscus sticks or hesitates. That could be the factor that causes the meniscus to position itself and then slip.

# III. Radiology of the Temporomandibular Joint

by Torsten Öberg

The subject "Radiology of the Temporomandibular Joint" is dealt with here mainly from my aspect as a clinician. For several years I have examined and treated patients with temporomandibular joint (TMJ) diseases in collaboration with Prof. *K.-Å. Omnell,* Head of the Department of Oral Radiology, School of Dentistry, Malmö, and his staff. I will present the methods for TMJ radiography used at this department.

Technical advances in TMJ radiology during the last ten years—not least of which was the introduction of tomography—together with increasing knowledge of the pathoanatomy of the TMJ diseases, have resulted in radiography becoming an important part of the examination and treatment of TMJ diseases.

A clinical and radiographic examination of 67-year-old persons living in southern Sweden has shown that there is a close relationship between TMJ pain and dysfunction and radiographically visible TMJ changes. TMJ pain and dysfunction were associated with condyle displacement and structural changes in the hard tissues. (*Lysell,* 1977[1]).

The radiographic examination of the TMJ naturally gives the most information about changes in the TMJ proper. But such an examination can also give some information on the status of the jaw muscles and the functional anatomy of the dentition, as well as on the biomechanical stress on the total stomatognathic system. Diseases affecting the TMJ proper may roughly be referred to the following groups:

Congenital defects
Postnatal growth disturbances
Tumors
Diseases caused by acute trauma
Condyle—disk displacement (subluxation)
Diseases due to loading
Microtraumatic arthritis
Remodeling and deviation in form
Arthrosis (Osteoarthritis)
RA and other connective tissue diseases
Arthritis and infection
Metabolic diseases
Miscellaneous

Only in a few of these diseases are the TMJ changes of such a character that radiography alone can establish a firm diagnosis. It should also be mentioned that absence of radiographically visible changes does not exclude disease of the joint. A firm diagnosis often requires inquiry into the patient's history, EMG and bite force measurements, as well as examinations by specialists such as rheumatologists, neurologists and otologists.

The important rule, that the radiographic examination of the TMJ should always be preceded by careful inquiry into the patient's history and by clinical examination, must be underlined. The clinical findings serve as a guide in the choice of radiological methods and in the interpretation of the radiographs.

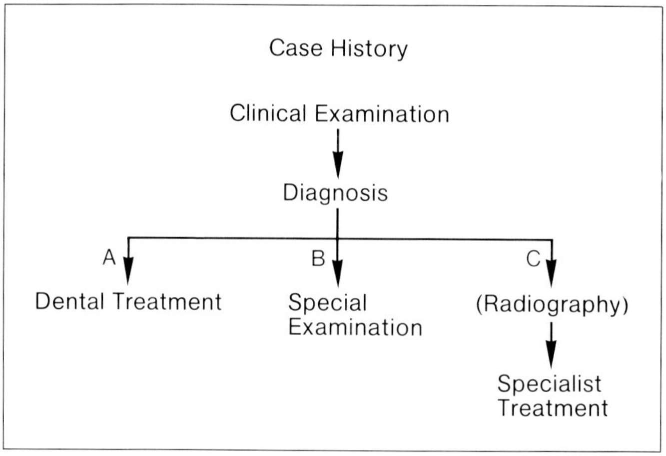


Fig. 1

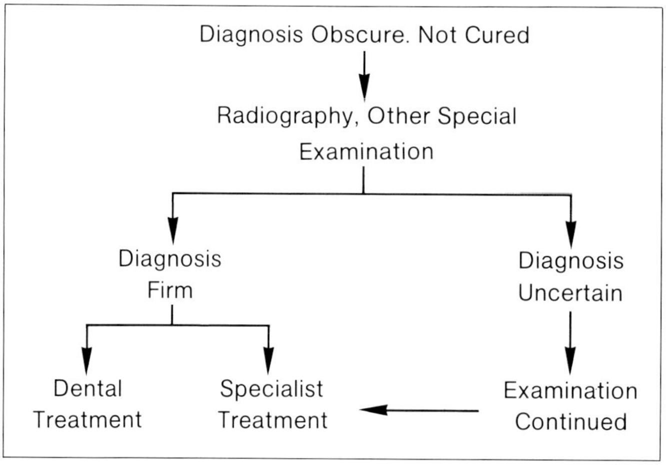


Fig. 2

The radiographic examination of the TMJ is mainly (1) for diagnostic purposes. But it is often helpful, (2) in determining the prognosis, (3) in the choice of therapeutic procedures, (4) for treatment planning, (5) to assess the effect of treatment and (6) to check the development of the disease.

In this discussion I will deal with the following: the position occupied by TMJ radiography in the examination and treatment of TMJ diseases, indications for TMJ radiography, some relevant parts of TMJ anatomy, examination technique, and finally, some case reports exemplifying the utilization of TMJ radiology.

## Examination and treatment of TMJ diseases

Figure 1 is to be understood as follows: A preliminary diagnosis is made on the basis of the case history and clinical examination. If the diagnosis is firm or probable and the disease probably benign, the dentist plans and initiates treatment (A). But if symptoms and clinical signs do not warrant a firm diagnosis, it is obscure or uncertain, there is need for special examinations (B). If there is reason to suspect some disease requiring urgent specialist treatment, such as an infectious arthritis or a fracture, the patient is referred to the hospital (C). Such cases are, however, relatively few. Before sending the patient to the hospital, an examination in a department of oral radiology may be indicated. In the group A patients, the simple conventional treatment procedures will occasionally fail to produce any cure or improvement. For these cases the diagnosis has to be reconsidered, and there is need for further examination.

From figure 2 it appears that special examinations are required for the groups of patients for which the diagnosis was obscure or uncertain (B), and for which the diagnosis is to be reconsidered. At present, the special examination normally used in my department is radiology of the TMJ followed by electromyography. Patients are also often referred to medical specialists for examination of suspected systemic diseases and for differential diagnostic purposes. These special examinations broaden the diagnostic basis and improve the possibility of arriving at a correct diagnosis. If such examinations give a firm diagnosis, treatment may be started, but if they do not, the investigation must be continued with supplementary methods. Further X-ray examination may later be indicated for treatment planning and following the course of the disease.

## Indications for TMJ radiography

Radiographic examination may be indicated if it is found that the patient has (1) a systemic disease capable of affecting the TMJ, such as rheumatoid arthritis RA, (2) swelling and other kinds of deformations in the region of the TMJ, (3) severe resting pain, pain on movement and tenderness to palpation, (4) joint stiffness and impaired mobility, (5) crepitations suggesting arthrosis, (6) acute trauma suspected of causing fracture or substantial soft tissue damage, (7) mandibular asymmetry or other abnormal position of the lower jaw suspected of being due to some disease of the joint, and finally (8) unusual functional anatomy of the dentition presumed to have an unfavorable effect on the relationship between the joint components. The indications are relative. If the joint symptoms are slight or moderate, and the preliminary diagnosis is firm or probable and the disease presumed benign, one may first wait and see what results from 3—4 weeks of "conservative" treatment. If no improvement occurs, the patient may be referred for radiography and other special examinations. (Fig. 1 and 2).

## TMJ anatomy

In the choice of examination techniques and in the interpretation of the radiographs the examiner must have a clear mental picture not only of the complicated anatomy of the joint, but also of nearby structures. When the TMJ stops growing at about age 20, there are considerable individual variations in the shape of the articulating joint components. Generally the components are gently rounded with smooth articulating surfaces. Their forms are well fitted to one another, from a functional point of view (*Oberg* and *Carlsson,* 1979[2]). In older age groups the joint surfaces can still be smooth and gently curved. In healthy adult joints the hard tissue outline against the overlying soft tissue is regular and evenly curved, (Fig. 3A), though a continuous internal remodeling in the compact bone layer is going on throughout life. This is

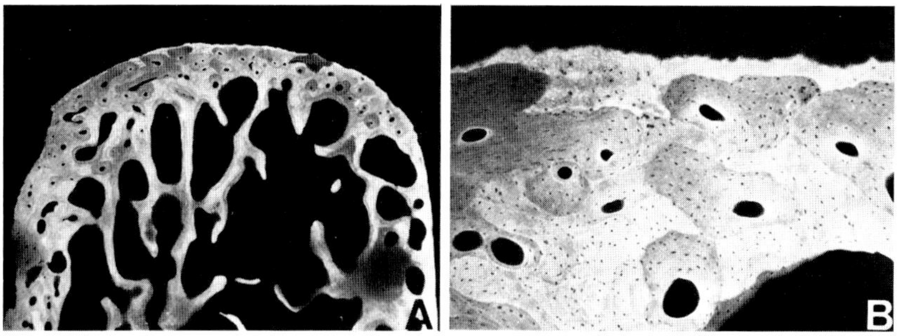


Fig. 3 A and B. A microradiograph of a ground section in the central part of the condyle from a 67-year-old individual. Section placed at right angles to longitudinal axis. The compact bone layer superior in the condyle in higher magnification in B.

obvious from the various degrees of mineralization in the osteons (B).

When interpreting routine radiographs it should be borne in mind that the hard tissue outline and the outline of the soft tissue surface are not parallel. This is due to the variation in the thickness of the soft tissue in different parts of the joint components (*Hansson, Öberg, Carlsson* and *Kopp,* 1977;[3] *Hansson* and *Nordstrom,* 1977;[4] *Bean, Omnell* and *Öberg,* 1977[5]).

The orientation of the condylar pole axis in relation to a frontal as well as a horizontal plane may vary widely. This has been shown by *Moffett* (1962)[6] and also by *Yale* and coworkers (1966)[7]. It is very important to take this variation into account in TMJ radiography.

The posterior part of the disk and adjoining part of the capsule consists of a sensitive loose connective tissue, rich in vessels and nerves. This tissue is very soft and flexible in order to permit condyle and disk to slide fairly far forward.

## Examination technique

Radiography of the TMJ should give the examiner a clear three-dimensional impression of the size, shape and structure of the joint, as well as an indication of its functional condition. The effect of treatment and the further course of a disease is best revealed if the radiographic examination is standardized in such a way that the projections are reproducible.

Radiographic examination of the TMJ can be static or dynamic. When static, images are obtained of the joint in well defined maxillomandibular relationships. The static examination can, however, also yield some information about the function of the joint. Dynamic examination means a continuous recording of the movements of the condyle. This method requires the use of an image-intensifier (fluoroscope) and preferably also documentation with the aid of cineradiography or videotape.

In routine methods it is mainly the osseous components that can be studied. Changes in these parts can, however, also give clues to the condition of the soft tissues. A certain amount of information about the soft tissues, particularly the thickness of the disk and the articular soft tissue layers, can be obtained by studying the relationships between the mineralized parts of the condyle and the temporal component, respectively, in different mandibular positions. Further knowledge of

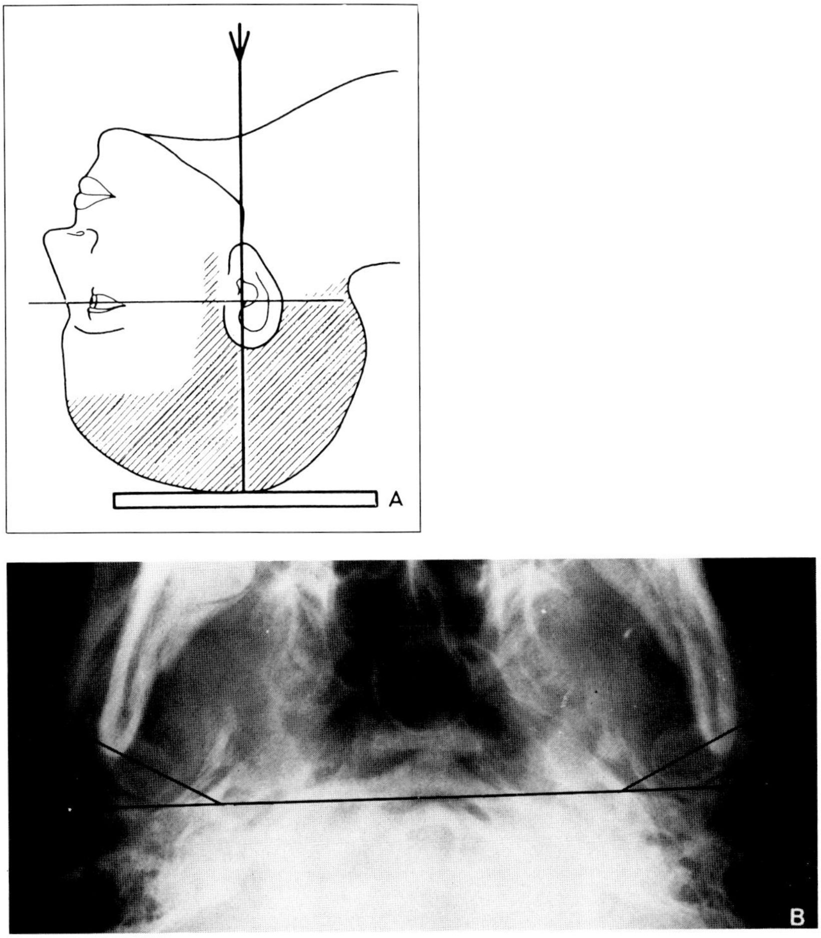


Fig. 4

A. Schematic drawing of the mento-vertical projection. (From *Omnell* and *Lysell*, 1974).
B. Mento-vertical radiograph. Before exposure, ear rods united with a bow are placed in the external auditory canals. The innermost part of each rod contains a lead ball. The line between the images of these balls is named the base line.

the condition of the soft tissues can be obtained by arthrography (*Norgaard* 1947,[8] *Toller* 1974,[9] *Blaschke* 1979[10]), or computerized tomography.
The examination routine used at the Department of Radiology at the School of Dentistry in Malmö will be described. For a detailed description see *Petersson* (1976).[11] It always includes the following projections in the order given: mento-vertical, transcranial and transmaxillary. In addition, tomography is now practically a routine procedure. Arthrography is used occasionally, but the technique is presently being refined. For computerized tomography we sometimes refer the patient to the University Hospital in Lund.

**Mento-vertical projection**

This projection (Fig. 4A) can yield valuable information on, among other things, fractures in the region of the joint and of hypo- or hyperplasia of the condyle.

The image also serves as a guide for the individualization of the transcranial projection. For this reason the angle betwen the projection of the respective longitudinal axes of the condyles in the film plane and base line is always measured (Fig. 4A).

**Transcranial projection**

In order to be able to obtain reproducible projections, the patient is examined sitting with the head fixed in a cephalostat that can be rotated in the horizontal plane in relation to the tube and the film, which are stationary (*Omnell & Petersson,* 1976).[13]

With the measured size of the condylar angle as a guide, the patient is rotated so that the central ray in the horizontal plane will run parallel to the longitudinal axis of the condyle (Fig. 5A). The angulation of the beam is 25° from above and is directed at right angles to the film (B).

The transcranial radiographs are taken routinely with the mandible in intercuspal position, postural position, and with the mouth wide open, all with the same film (Fig. 6). Notice how the condyle normally "drops" somewhat in infero-anterior direction on its way from the intercuspal position to postural position.

It should be emphasized that these radiographs give information mainly about the bone structures in the lateral parts of the joint.

**Transmaxillary projection**

With the patient sitting, the occlusal plane is placed horizontally. The patient's mouth is open so that the condyles, if possible, have translated below the eminence. The central ray is directed just below the infraorbital foramen and passes through the maxillary sinus on the other side falling on the film at an angle of 90° (Fig. 7A). To secure an image with a minimum of superimpositions from the mastoid process, *Petersson* and *Nanthaviroj* (1975)[14] found that the horizontal angulation of the central ray to the midsagittal plane should be about 40°. The optimum vertical angulation was found to be + 10°. The radiograph gives a view of the condyle in a medio-lateral plane and, under favorable circumstances, also of the lower part of the tubercle (Fig. 7B).

**Tomographic examination**

In tomography a predetermined layer of an object is brought out more distinctly, while structures before and behind the layer are blurred or eliminated.

In Malmö, the tomographic examination is performed with a Philips Polytome, utilizing the hypocycloidal movement. The patient's head is oriented and fixed in roughly the same way as in the individualized technique for transcranial projection. The examination is usually performed with the tomographic layer perpendicular or parallel to the longitudinal axis of the condyle. A method for standardized mento-vertical horizontal tomography has also been devised in Malmö by *Faivovich* and *Omnell* (1977)[15].

Since the development of a cassette for simultaneous tomography (Siemens Simultan), in which one exposure shows five sections at different levels of the joint (*Petersson,* 1979[16]), tomography is now almost a routine procedure in our radiographic examination.

The sets of radiographs in Figure 8 (from *Omnell* and *Petersson,* 1976[13]) illustrate the value of tomography in determining the relationship between the joint components.

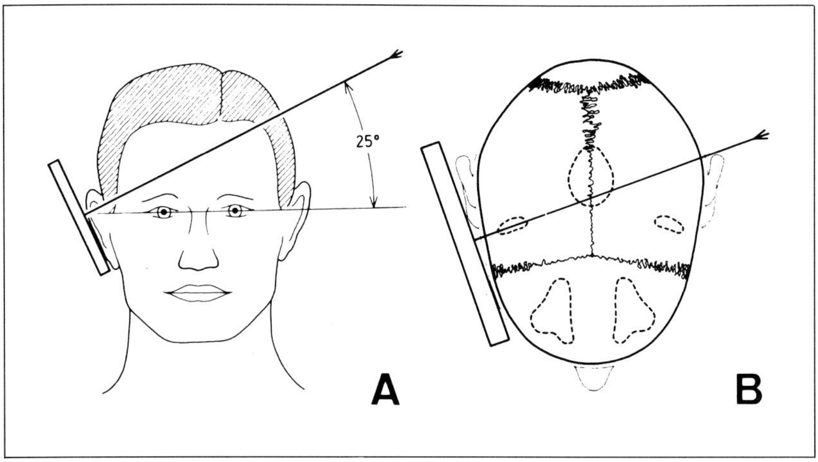


Fig. 5 Schematic drawings of individualized transcranial projection. (From *Omnell* and *Lysell*, 1974).

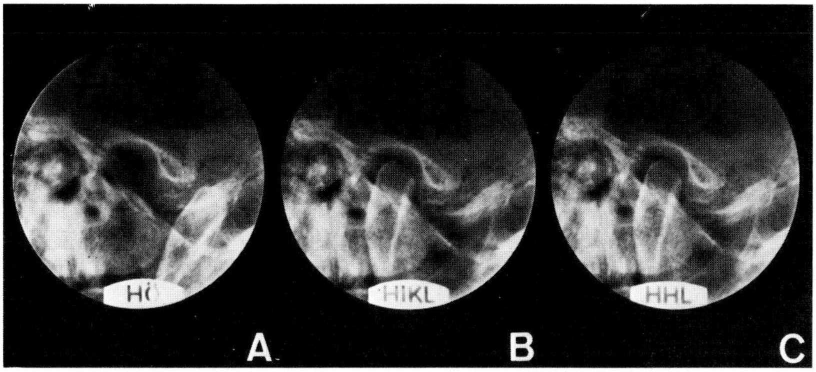


Fig. 6 Individualized transcranial radiographs of right TMJ in maximal opening, A (HO), intercuspal position, B (HIKL) and postural position (HHL).

A—F: Radiographs of a right TMJ resulting from standard positioning (A), individualized positioning (B) and tomography with the plane of sectioning perpendicular to the long axis of the condyle (C—F). C and D represent the lateral, E the central and F the medial third of the joint. The same condyle to fossa relation occurs in all positions of the joint. G—J: This set of tomograms from another patient illustrates a situation where the condyle to fossa relation varies from lateral (G) to the medial (J) third of the joint. Tomography can also visualize structural changes not demonstrable in conventional radiographs.

*Peterson* (1976)[11] has compared the information obtainable with different techniques. He concluded that individualized trans-

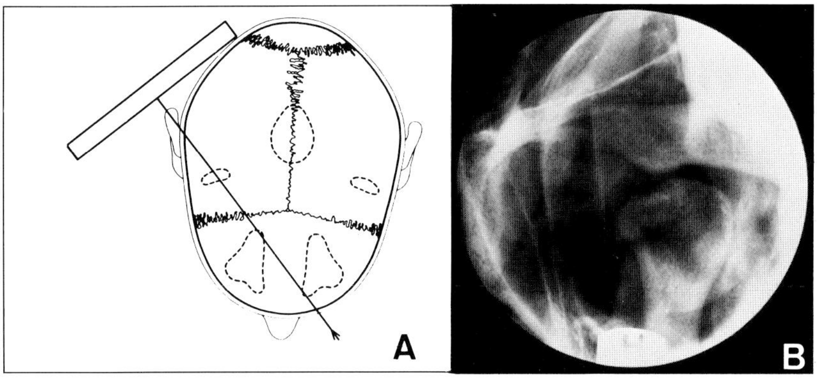


Fig. 7

A. Schematic drawing of the transmaxillary projection. (From *Omnell* and *Lysell*, 1974).
B. Transmaxillary radiograph of right TMJ.

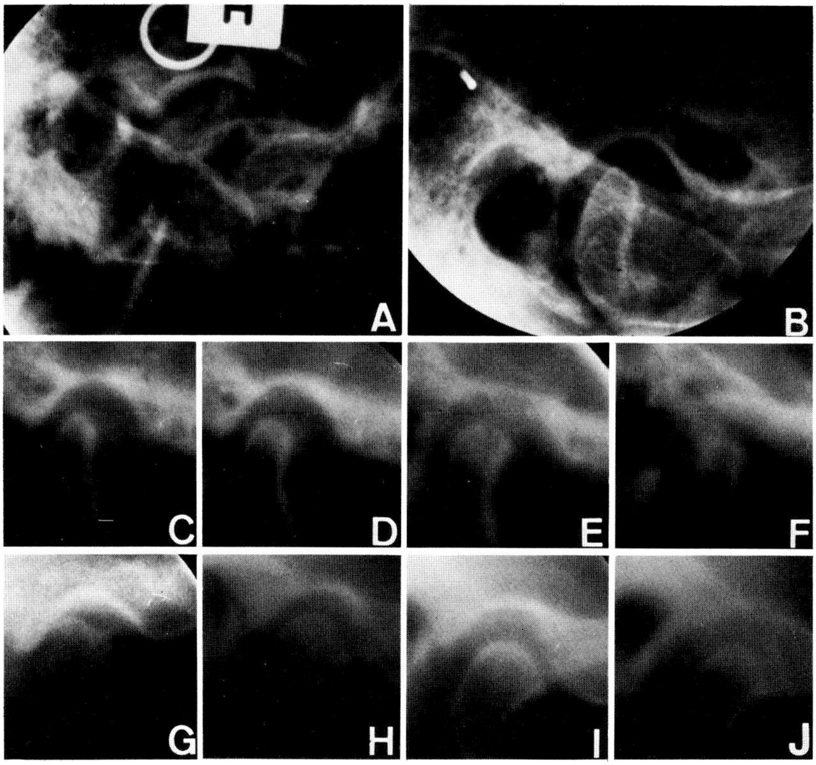


Fig. 8

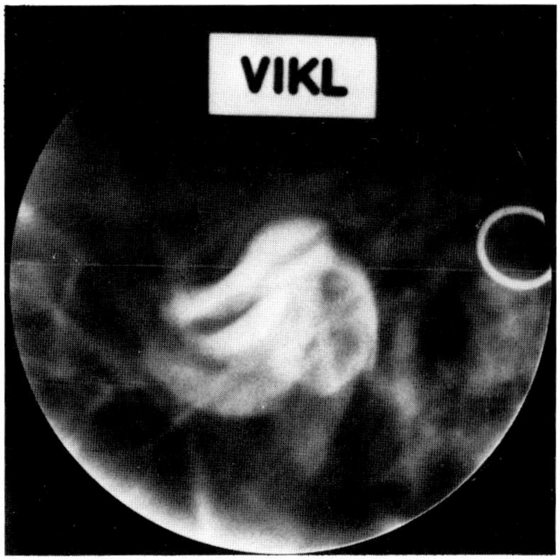


Fig. 9 Arthrogram of left TMJ, intercuspal position. Transcranial projection. The contrast medium has been injected to the upper joint compartment. There is a perforation of the disc as the medium has flowed into the lower compartment.

cranial projection is better than standard transcranial projection for revealing structural changes, and that the former gives more information about structural changes than does the transmaxillary projection. However, the transmaxillary technique contributes substantially to the total information available, since this method can visualize things which other methods cannot. He also stated that the transcranial projection with the standard technique and the individualized technique are unreliable regarding the relationship between the condyle and the temporal component in intercuspal position, and that tomography, the method of choice for radiography of the TMJ, should be combined with the individualized transcranial projection and the transmaxillary projection, to obtain maximum information.

In most cases, I supplement the routine examination of the TMJ with an orthopantomogram.

**Arthrography**

Arthrography, a roentgenographic examination after injection of a contrast medium into the joint spaces of the TMJ, may be used for demonstrating perforations of the disk or capsule (Fig. 9). This method can also reveal condyle-disk displacement (subluxation) in the joint, as well as show the thickness of the soft tissue on the condyle and the fossa.

Radiographs of the TMJ give us information about: (1) the relationship between the articulating components in different positions, (2) the size and form of the components and (3) the structure of compact bone, spongy bone and soft tissues. Structural changes in the hard tissue which are often seen are: erosions, flattenings, osteophytes and sclerosis.

The various types of changes were examplified in case reports at the Symposium. A few of them will be presented here in a limited form.

## Case reports

As mentioned in the introduction, the diseases of the TMJ may roughly be assigned to the following groups:

### Congenital defects

The transcranial radiograph disclosed nothing remarkable, but the transmaxillary picture revealed a bifid condyle and also adaptive changes in the articular tubercle causing locking and clicking. For the diagnosis in this case the radiological findings were decisive.

### Postnatal growth disturbances

Postnatal growth disturbances may either be due to overdevelopment or underdevelopment. The condyle as well as the temporal component may be affected. An example of overdevelopment is unilateral hyperplasia of the mandibular condylar process, the etiology of which is obscure. Profile and full-face radiographs showed asymmetries of the facial skeleton and radiographs of the TMJ showed the enlarged condyle.

### Tumors

Tumors in the TMJ are unusual, but the possibility of a tumor should not be forgotten in the examination of patients with pain and dysfunction of this region.

A 63-year-old man came to the clinic because of pain in the region of his left TMJ and difficulty in opening his mouth. The symptoms had suddenly begun 14 days previously, when the patient had heard a snapping noise in the joint. Examination showed tenderness to palpation of the masticatory muscles and the TMJ on the left side, and only slight mobility of the condyle. The orthopantomogram disclosed a large radiolucent area in the region of the left condylar process extending into the posteromedial part of the ramus. (Fig. 10A). Tomographic examination showed that only the lateral third of the condyle and a thin arc of bone of the mandibular neck remained (B). In the neck area a fracture was found and explained the sudden onset of pain. Although generalized skeletal involvement was excluded, laboratory findings were considered consistent with a diagnosis of multiple myeloma.

### Diseases due to acute trauma

The consequences of an acute trauma, direct or indirect, against the TMJ may be soft tissue lesions, dislocation (luxation) and fracture, separately or in combination. Besides the initial tissue changes with accompanying symptoms, the injury, especially when severe, may be followed by obstinate or irreversible sequelae. In most cases the radiographic examination of the TMJ is important. Case histories suggest that an acute trauma may be a fairly common cause of symptoms from the TMJ. (*Carlsson, Kopp* and *Oberg,* 1979)[18].

Even a mild injury such as a *contusion* of the soft tissue of the TMJ, following a trivial trauma, is usually sufficient to cause edema of the posterior, loose part of the disk and of the capsule, as well as synovitis and sometimes a serious effusion. The acute phase is characterized by, among other things, pain and tenderness to palpation. The inflammatory reaction results in loss of firm contact between the molars on the affected side. There is a markedly greater radiographic distance between the roof of the fossa and the condyle in the tomogram of the affected side, reflecting the edema and hydrarthrosis.

In more severe lesions, such as shearing, crushing and dislocation of the disk or avulsion of the capsule, the diagnosis may be facilitated by arthrography (Fig. 9). Trau-

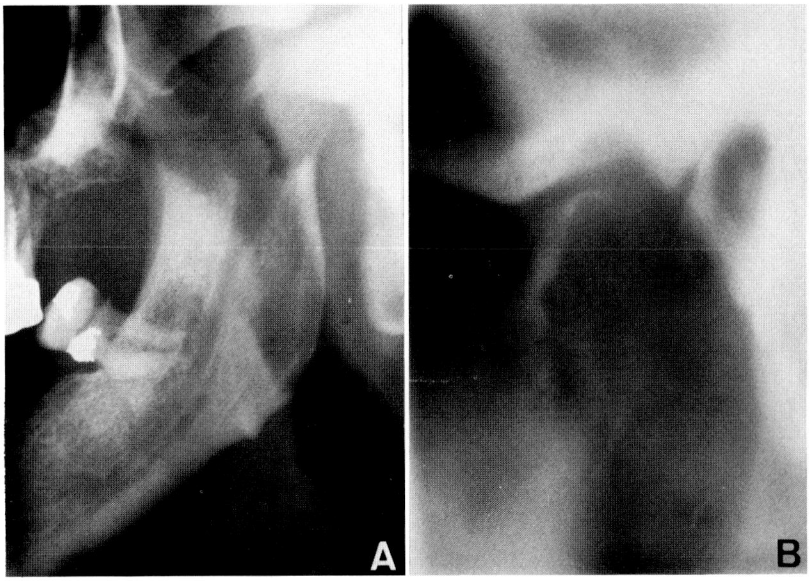


Fig. 10

A. Left part of orthopantomogram.
B. Tomogram of left TMJ. (From *Jagger, Helkimo* and *Carlsson*, 1978).

matic injuries may be followed by cicatrical contractions, adhesions and even fibrous or bony ankylosis of the joint.

Fracture of the condylar process is common. Usually, the fracture is accompanied by more or less severe damage to the capsule and the disk. In the acute phase this invariably causes traumatic arthritis with the characteristics described earlier.

The radiographic examination is decisive for the diagnosis of a fracture—especially if it is a question of a nondisplaced fracture.

### Condyle-disk displacement (subluxation)

According to my opinion, a condyle-disk displacement is a subluxation, that is, an incomplete or partial dislocation.

The most common subluxation of the TMJ is obviously when the condyle, in the intercuspal position is pressed backward at the same time as the disk is rotated anteriorly, so that the superior part of the condyle is situated behind the posterior dense and thick part of the disk. This can cause locking of the condyle during mouth opening, as well as a repeated trauma against the posterior loose soft tissue of the joint.

We have made a clinical-radiological investigation on 10 patients with a marked "locking"/clicking of the TMJ during opening movement of the mouth (*Nanthaviroj, Omnell, Randow* and *Öberg,* 1976[19]). The most consistent result, obtained with tomography, revealed that the distance between the mineralized parts of the condyle and the temporal component was invariably larger just before, rather than just after, "locking"/-clicking. This indicated a soft tissue obstacle, which might be due to a subluxation, or a soft tissue thickening in the condyle, or the articular tubercle, or a combination of both.

## Diseases due to loading

Probably the most common group of diseases which affect temporomandibular joints and muscles—and which also frequently occur in the teeth and periodontium —is a group which may be categorized as diseases due to loading. Biomechanical loading during function and parafunction plays an important or dominating role in the development of these tissue changes (*Hansson,* 1979[20]). "Loading diseases" of the TMJ proper are microtraumatic arthritis and advanced remodeling, deviation in form and arthrosis. These diseases may appear isolated or combined.

*Microtraumatic arthritis.* — Repeated compression and tension of the peripheral loose part of the disk and of the joint capsule may cause an inflammatory reaction. The condyle can then be displaced forwards and downwards as after an acute trauma.

*Remodeling, deviation in form* and *arthrosis.* — Microtraumatization of the articulating components can stimulate remodeling of the tissue layers to such an extent that it results in a deviation in form of the components which may interfere with joint function. Eventually the changes may progress to pathological conditions, such as arthrosis. Such changes are very common in adults (*Hansson,* 1979[20]).

From one of our autopsy studies I will give an example of a joint with advanced hard and soft tissue remodeling and deviation in form, Fig. 11.

Laterally, on the posterior slope of the articular tubercle, there is a remarkable elevation of the surface (A). The elevation is situated opposite a flattened protruberance, laterally and antero-superiorly on the condyle (B). Note also the humplike shape of the superior part. Despite the changes in form, the articulating surfaces don't exhibit any macroscopic signs of arthrotic lesions. The disk has been passively adapted to the contours of the other two components. From the pictures (A, C) it is obvious that the lateral elevation on the tubercle was mainly due to a thickening of the soft tissues. Also in the under-lying hard tissues a deviation in form due to a progressive remodeling was seen. However, in the central part of this elevation there was a regressive remodeling with a perforation of the compact bone layer in the lateral part. A sagittal tomogram showed the so-called erosive lesion in the posterior slope of the articular tubercle (D). This illustrates well that the diagnosis of arthrosis cannot be made solely on the basis of such hard tissue changes found in the roentgenograms.

This 65-year-old woman had an old complete denture which gave insufficient stabilization to the lower jaw. The patient showed resting pain in the right TMJ and temporal region, pain in the joint when biting hard in ICP, and crepitation and pain on movement. Transcranial radiographs indicated deviation in form and a displaced condyle (Fig. 12A). The tomographic examination showed an almost normal picture in the medial part of the joint (B). The tomogram from the lateral part of the joint revealed the characteristic deviation in form of the condyle (C). Practically no space existed between the mineralized parts of the condyle and fossa. Sclerosis in the fossa (postero-superiorly) indicated an arthrotic lesion in the lateral wall of the fossa and a perforation of the disk.

By means of a temporary splinting, the unfavorable biomechanical load of the arthrotic area had been removed. This was verified by the widened space between condyle and fossa (D). The pain disappeared within two days.

## RA and other connective tissue diseases

Involvement of the TMJs in patients with RA is common (*Carlsson, Kopp* and *Öberg,*

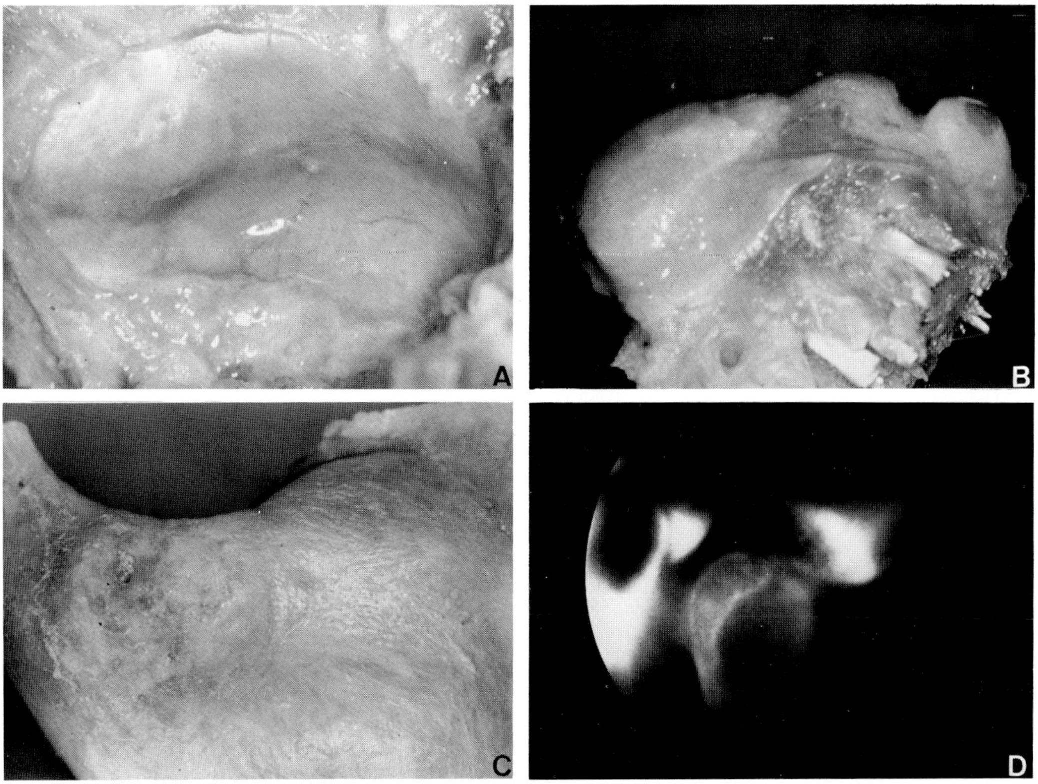


Fig. 11 TMJ with fairly advanced deviation in form (DIF) due to hard and soft tissue remodeling.

A. Temporal component, anterior upwards, lateral to the left.
B. Condyle, anterior view, lateral to the left.
C. Temporal component after removal of the soft tissues.
D. "Transcranial" tomogram from the lateral part of the joint.

1979[18]). Sooner or later more than 40 % of these persons seem to get clinical symptoms in the TMJ. By means of radiography alone it is difficult or impossible to diagnose changes in the TMJ due to RA. This holds true, at any rate, for the early stages of the disease. Probably erosive changes such as "a hollowing out and irregular destruction" of the joint components, particularly of the tubercle, are the most characteristic alterations in RA, but such changes are seldom seen during the first 5 years of the disease.

## Arthritis and infection

Infectious diseases are sometimes accompanied or followed by arthritis. The frequency of septic joint diseases has decreased substantially since the advent of antibiotics. On the other hand, various form of aseptic arthritis have appeared in which there is reason to suspect a causal connection between infection and arthritis. An acute septic arthritis usually affects only one joint. The onset is most often acute with severe

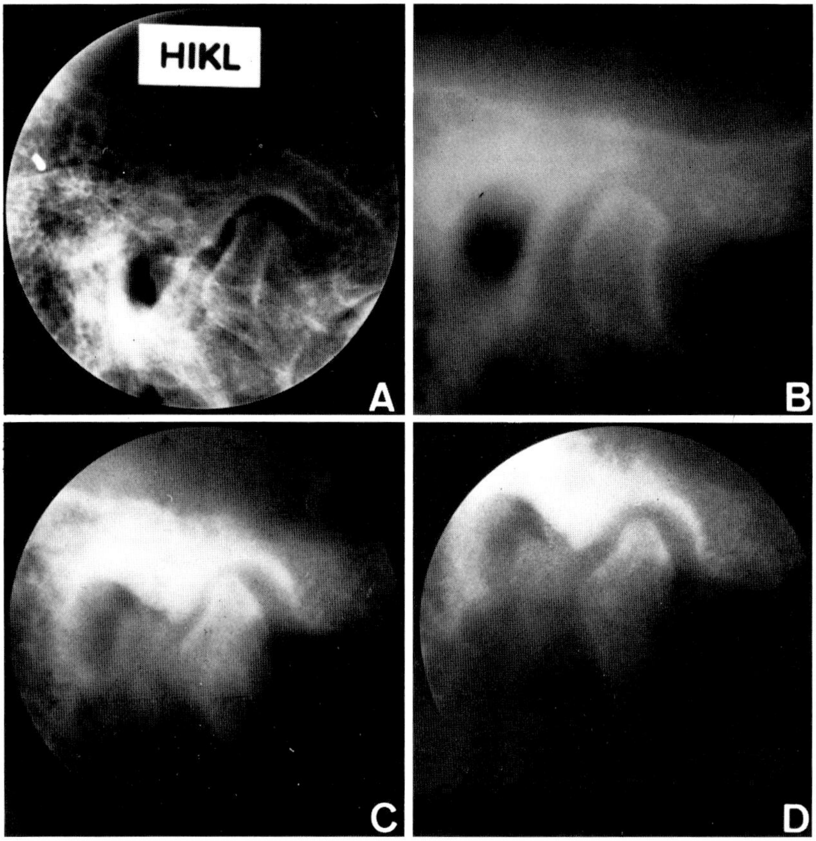


Fig. 12 Radiographs of right TMJ with a local arthrosis laterally in the joint.

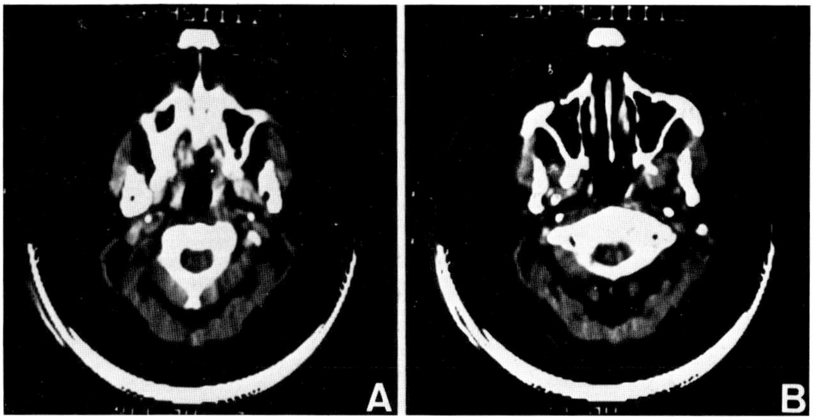


Fig. 13 Computerized tomograms on two different horizontal levels showing hard tissue exophytes from the pterygoid lamina and from the medial side of the inferior part of the mandibular ramus, on the right side.

resting pain and pain on movement, swelling, increased temperature, reddening and tenderness of the joint to palpation.
No destructive changes are radiographically demonstrable during the first week. But in the TMJ, hydrops and edema maintain an antero-inferior position of the condyle—visible in the radiograph—also when the mouth is closed.

### Miscellaneous

The radiographic examination, shown in Figure 13, revealed the cause of a markedly reduced mobility of the mandible in a 57-year-old man, who was referred to the clinic because of difficulty in opening his mouth. For 20 years he had had a right-sided trigeminal neuralgia. During the last ten years about 30 injections of alcohol and local anesthetics had been given in the region of the mandibular foramen to block the mandibular and the lingual nerve. The last alcohol injection was six years ago. At the beginning he had varying, but during the last five years constantly increasing difficulty in opening, making odontological treatment troublesome. The clinical examination revealed a maximal opening capacity of the mouth of 17 mm. In the jaw muscles available to palpation no tenderness was found. There was impaired mobility in the temporomandibular joints, but a "joint play" was noted and a translatory movement palpated in both joints. These findings indicated a non-articular cause of the severely impaired mouth opening capacity. Transcranial radiography also argued against the possibility that the reduced mandibular mobility was arthrogenic. Both a frontal radiograph and the orthopantomogram showed the radiopacity to be stronger medially to the ramus on the right side than on the left. The mento-vertical tomograms showed hard tissue exophytes from the pterygoid lamina and from the medial side of the inferior part of the mandibular ramus, on the right side. Computerized tomograms gave the same result as the conventional tomograms. Obviously, a fibrous dysplasia of the medial pterygoid muscle due to the injection had resulted in a stimulation of bone formation at the muscle attachments.

### References


1. *Lysell, L.*
Epidemiologic-roentgen diagnostic study on teeth, jaws and temporomandibular joints in 67-year-old people in Dalby, Sweden. Thesis. University of Lund, Malmö, Sweden. 1977

2. *Öberg, T. & Carlsson, G. E.*
Macroscopic and microscopic anatomy of the temporomandibular joint. In Temporomandibular Joint, Function and Dysfunction. Eds. George A. Zarb & Gunnar E. Carlsson. Munksgaard, Copenhagen. The C. V. Mosby Company, St. Louis, Missouri. 1979

3. *Hansson, T., Öberg, T., Carlsson, G. E. & Kopp, S.*
Thickness of the soft tissue layers and the articular disk in the temporomandibular joint. Acta Odontol. Scand. 35: 77—83. 1977

4. *Hansson, T. & Nordstrom, B.*
Thickness of the soft tissue layers and the articular disc in the temporomandibular joint with deviations in form. Acta Odontol. Scand. 35: 281–288. 1977

5. *Bean, L. R., Omnell, K.-A. & Öberg, T.*
Comparison between radiologic observations and macroscopic tissue changes in temporomandibular joints. Dentomaxillofac. Radiol. 6: 90—106. 1977

6. *Moffett, B.*
The temporomandibular joint. In Complete Denture Prosthodontics. Eds. Sharry, J. J. McGraw-Hill, New York, Toronto, London. 1962

7. *Yale, S., Allison, B. D. & Hauptfuehrer, J. D.*
An epidemiological assessment of mandibular condyle morphology. Oral Surg. 21: 169–177. 1966

8. *Norgaard, F.*
Temporomandibular arthrography. Munksgaard, Copenhagen. 1947

9. *Toller, P. A.*
Temporomandibular arthropathy. Proc. Roy. Soc. Med. 67: 153—159. 1974

10. *Blaschke, D.*
Arthrography of the temporomandibular joint. In Temporomandibular Joint Problems, Biologic Diagnosis and Treatment. Eds. W. K. Solberg and G. T. Clark. Quintessence Publishing Co., Inc. Berlin 1980.

11. *Petersson, A.*
Radiography of the temporomandibular joint. A comparison of information obtained from different radiographic techniques. Thesis. University of Lund, Malmö, Sweden. 1976

12. *Omnell, K.-A. & Lysell, L.*
Rontgendiagnostik. In Bidfunktion/Bettfysiologi II. Eds. Willy Krogh-Poulsen & Ole Carlsen, Munksgaard, Copenhagen. 1974

13. *Omnell, K.-A. & Petersson, A.*
Radiography of the temporomandibular joint utilizing oblique lateral transcranial projection. Odontol. Revy 27: 77—92. 1976

14. *Petersson, A. & Nanthaviroj, S.*
Radiography of the temporomandibular joint utilizing the transmaxillary projection. Dentomaxillofac. Radiol 4: 76—83. 1975

15. *Faivovich, G. & Omnell, K.-A.*
Axial tomography of the temporomandibular joint using hypocycloidal movement of tube and film. Dentomaxillofac. Radiol 6: 7—16. 1977

16. *Petersson, A.*
Personal communication. Department of Oral Radiology, University of Lund, School of Dentistry, S—214 21 Malmö, Sweden. 1979

17. *Jagger, R. G., Helkimo, M. & Carlsson, G. E.*
Multiple myeloma involving the temporomandibular joint: report of case. J Oral Surg 36. 557–559. 1978

18. *Carlsson, G. E., Kopp, S. & Öberg, T.*
Arthritis and allied diseases of the temporomandibular joint. In Temporomandibular Joint, Function and Dysfunction. Eds. *George A. Zarb & Gunnar E. Carlsson.* Munksgaard, Copenhagen. The C. V. Mosby Company, St. Louis, Missouri. 1979

19. *Nanthaviroj, S., Omnell, K.-A., Randow, K. & Öberg, T.*
Clicking and temporary "locking" in the temporomandibular joint. A clinical, radiographical and electromyographical study. Dentomaxillofac. Radiol 5: 33—38. 1976

20. *Hansson, T.*
TMJ changes related to dental occlusion. In Temporomandibular Joint Problems, Biologic diagnosis and treatment. Eds. W. K. Solberg and G. T. Clark. Quintessence Publishing Co., Inc. Berlin 1980.

# Discussion

Discussant: Donald Blaschke

*Dr. Blaschke*

Speaking as a Oral Radiologist I want to tell you that I learned much from this lecture. For those of you who are not familiar with Dr. *Öberg's* University at Lund, Sweden, I can tell you that it's world renowned in TMJ radiology. Drs. *Omnell* and *Petersson,* of that department have done a lot to improve our knowledge of TMJ radiology. One reason for this is their use of the polytome. We saw many beautiful, multidirectional tomographic pictures on the screen just recently. Not very many dental schools in this country could afford such a machine and use it specifically for TMJ radiology. Besides the clinical expertise in the TMJ clinics at Lund, they also have exceptional equipment.

I would like to make a couple of comments on the basic aspects of radiology of the TMJ in terms of the general dentist or specialist. Dr. *Moffett* alluded to this earlier, and Dr. *Öberg* commented on it. When are TMJ radiographs really indicated? My position is that, anytime a joint is symptomatic, joint radiographs should be taken. We may even take TMJ radiographs on an asymptomatic joint if, on the basis of other projections, we have evidence to indicate that there may be a TMJ abnormality. For example, in our series of TMJ radiographs, we first look at a panoramic for an overall evaluation of the TMJ. This might then be followed by transcranial projections or tomograms.

I also want to make the point that many of the projections just demonstrated are applicable to the private dental office; especially the transcranial projection. The transmaxillary projection which Dr. *Petersson* has dealt with and the transpharyngeal or infracranial projection can all be made with a standard dental X-ray machine. They are made with a standard dental X-ray machine and a 5 x 7 cassette which can easily be held by the patient. I think that many practitioners don't take advantage of these projections, though they really involve very little cost and can be tremendously helpful.

Keep in mind the type of information you can get from a TMJ radiograph. Panoramic radiographs we use only for gross appreciation of condylar deformities, fractures; that sort of thing. I would say the transcranial is probably the most practical projection for the people in this room who are concerned with dental occlusion problems and structural changes on the articulating surfaces. However, transcranial radiography, as Dr. *Öberg* alluded, is not very helpful in definitively determining condyle relation within the fossa. Transcranial radiographs, which only project the lateral aspect of the condyle, are not good for demonstrating joint bony relationships. Tomography, I concur, is the way to study joint relationships. But I don't want to steer any clinician away from transcranial radiography, however, since it projects joint articulating structural abnormalities. For example, subcondylar sclerosis, flattening, and osteophytes can all be seen beautifully on this projection.

I would like to ask Dr. *Öberg* a question regarding "corrections" for both transcranials and tomography. Most oral radiologists and many TMJ specialists understand that we rotate the head about 20° toward the side of involvement when we are making either one of those projections. There has been some controversy as to whether or not we should individualize each patient by first taking a submental-vertex radiograph. Do you feel that it is necessary to take the time and the expense of the submental-vertex projection for individually lining up each condyle to the central X-ray beam?

*Dr. Öberg*

Dr. *Omnell* and Dr. *Petersson* have made an investigation which clearly shows that you can derive much more information from the individualized than from the standardized projection. Although it doesn't take much time for this projection, I think it would be more worthwhile for a general practitioner to take a standard view transcranial radiograph for a gross overview of the condylar process. The individualized projection is really only for detailed appreciation.

*Dr. Solberg*

Dr. *Petersson*, could you comment?

*Dr. Arne Petersson* (Sweden)

In Sweden the general practitioner never takes TMJ radiographs himself. If I were a general practitioner here I think I would take the standardized projection.

*Dr. Solberg*

What type of view would you recommend for a patient who walks in the door with fairly clear cut pain and dysfunction around the temporomandibular area? Dr. *Öberg* has suggested, I believe, that at least a short period of conservative treatment be made prior to the time that you do joint views.

*Dr. Petersson*

I agree. It should be stressed that you can never trust a transcranial projection for showing joint relationships; it's just for showing structural changes in the bone.

*Dr. Solberg*

So the condyle-temporal bone relationship, viewed in the sagittal plane is not very reliable with the transcranial projection. When do you take the orthopantomograph?

*Dr. Petersson*

We take it on all patients, to examine the entire mandible and teeth.

*Dr. Laskin*

Dr. *Öberg* mentioned that both *Yale* and his co-workers and *Moffett* have shown that there is considerable variation, not only in the horizontal angle of the condyle, but in the vertical angle. You can have a negative or positive angle, or no angle. Why are you compensating only for the horizontal angle, which seems to be less variable than the vertical change?

*Dr. Blaschke*

In transcranial radiography other considerations are paramount. The vertical angulation is basically designed to clear the petrous ridge on the side of the TMJ in question. We saw many transcranial radiographs with a dense bony oblique ridge running through the neck of the condyle. The 25° vertical caudal angulation is designed to clear that ridge from the condylar head. If you go very much below this angulation, say 10 to 15°, the ridge will come right across the condylar head. Conversely the more you increase that angulation the more you cause distortion of the condylar head and the fossa. Since one is projecting only the lateral aspect of the joint, I just don't think that it is worth compensating for. As far as tomography goes the sections are so thin with the polytome, only one or two millimeters, that it is just not necessary to perfectly produce a longitudinal condyle image to get discreet cortical outlines. At any rate the vertical angle discrepancy is not great. Dr. *Yale*'s study (1966) showed an average vertical angle of 5° in condyles; not markedly different from the horizontal X-ray beam used in tomography.

*Dr. Solberg*

I would like to move on to one point that I thought was very startling and that Dr. *Öberg* showed so beautifully. That is, what happens to the condylar shape, to an altered condyle once you start treatment? I believe you showed that the form tends to change under occlusal treatment, or different occlusal loading. Is that correct?

*Dr. Öberg*

It is fairly common that you can have some articular hard tissue lesions, also lesions in the condyle, and still maintain intact soft tissue. Perhaps if it occurs fairly early and if you can take away the unfavorable biomechanical stress, you have the possibility of this changing back without developing an arthrotic lesion. So this is, I think, a reason that we should try to have a good stabilization of the lower jaw throughout life. Then we shall not have the biomechanical stresses which induce remodeling processes in the hard and soft tissue, which can lead to deviations in form and functional disturbances, and finally turn in to an arthrotic lesion.

*Dr. Solberg*

I wonder if any of the other speakers have any comments on condyle form or remodeling following treatment?

*Dr. Mahan*

In the usual cases with degenerative arthritis, the patient experiences the sudden onset or the gradual onset of pain and in 8 months it goes away. *Toller* demonstrated some evidence that in 70% of his 130 cases, the pain goes away in 8 months. There is other evidence that the degenerated surfaces in the TMJ joints, in degenerative arthritis, will "heal" or reossify.

*Dr. Öberg*

I must say that in Dr. *Toller*'s investigations, only the TMJ condyle was examined. It is uncommon that you find an arthrotic lesion in the condyle. It is in the temporal component and in the disc you have arthrotic lesions. So I think he has missed much. It is such subarticular remodeling processes in the hard tissue which he has named arthritis.

*Dr. Mahan*

I was calling it degenerative arthritis; he called it TMJ arthrosis, but he has the radiographs that have shown healing. We see the same thing in degenerative arthritis so that even without therapy a good number of them look quite normal within a year and a half. We have seen joints with condylar shaves or condylotomies and two years later those condyles look normal.

*Dr. Blaschke*

I would like to ask Dr. *Öberg* if, at his University, deviations in form or prearthrotic lesions on the condyle head are identifiable by polytomography on a routine basis. We saw a definite deviation in form on a cadaver specimen here, but can your radiologist routinely diagnose these prearthrotic bony lesions?

*Dr. Öberg*

Yes, they are capable of doing this.

*Dr. Rick Temple* (Palm Springs, California)

Regarding computerized tomography, what are your indications, what views do you use and what are the thicknesses of your cuts?

*Dr. Öberg*

We have very little experience with this method. We have no such equipment in our dental school. But, we are sending some of our patients to the University Hospital in Lund to have them examined. Since there is also the possibility to see the muscles and the soft tissues (for example, the disc), I think this will be very valuable for us later on for diagnosis and treatment of TMJ joint problems.

*Dr. Solberg*

There is time for one question.

*Dr. Glenn Clark*

Dr. *Öberg*, you showed remodeling of the TMJ using a splint appliance and you said the patient was only wearing that splint at night. It seems to me that 12 hours of wearing a splint and 12 hours of not wearing it would be counterproductive. Why don't the patients wear the splint full-time?

*Dr. Öberg*

Yes, in this patient, as part of the primary treatment, we also eliminated the occlusal interferences. This permanent change in the occlusion could give such a result. Then the patient wears the splint during the night. When you take away this biomechanical loading during the night, instruct the patient to relax during the day, and take away the occlusal interferences, I think it is enough to have the patient wear the splint only in the night.

*Dr. Solberg*

One last question.

*Dr. Knud Flygenring* (Northridge, California)

It has been alluded to throughout this presentation that there is some value in the panoramic radiograph. It pleases me that we can get some suspicion of something happening by a panoramic radiograph taken in a standard way. Some techniques have been developed that do a specific TMJ projection and in this way only have the joint present on the film. This is a transcranial projection. Could you give an evaluation ot the value of this specific technique?

*Dr. Blaschke*

We use a panoramic projection in the standard way for what we feel is very adequate visualization of the condylar process, although we don't see the articular fossa or sometimes the articulating surface of the condyle. We feel that if there are gross abnormalities, something which catches our eye, we can certainly go to the other projections. We make a panoramic projection in a series of TMJ views, so that's the reason we don't do these specialized panoramic views. Various manufacturers of panoramic X-ray machines provide detailed technical instructions on how to make open mouth TMJ views. Some of them are exceptional. Again, we have access to specialized TMJ radiographs which are superior to panoramics. I must advise the group that panoramic radiography usually projects the condyle in an oblique fashion, not in a cross-sectional view. Very often that makes very subtle abnormalities hard to see. But, again, for a gross appreciation, some of these techniques are pretty good.

*Dr. Öberg*

I think, for the general practitioner, that's one of the questions that came up—what can we use out in practice?

*Dr. Blaschke*

I dont't think it would be very difficult to work on a few patients with your dental assistant or your technician. Just practice a few of the transcranial or special panoramic projections and they'll get better. I think that it would be a good thing for private practice.

# IV. Arthrography of the Temporomandibular Joint

by Donald D. Blaschke

## Introduction

I am very honored to be in this program, especially as part of such a distinguished panel, and I am especially pleased to speak to the Newport Harbor Academy of Dentistry and the UCLA Continuing Education Program. I would like to mention at the start that I am indebted to Dr. *Clyde Wilkes* of Minneapolis for demonstrating to me his technique in performing TMJ arthrography. In my early practice of temporomandibular arthrography, I relied heavily on Dr. *Wilkes'* techniques and concepts of interpretation. Dr. *William Solberg* should also receive much of the credit for UCLA's TMJ arthrographic service. There have been occasional spells during which I have been discouraged with the procedure and *Bill* has given me the encouragement to keep at it.

## General concept and goal of TMJ arthrography

The basic concept of arthrography of any joint is to artificially change the radiographic density of the joint spaces, thereby providing contrast to the soft tissues of the joint. This change in density is almost always in the direction of making the spaces radiopaque relative to the adjacent soft tissues. The procedure is accomplished by injecting into the joint spaces a water soluble, tissue compatible, radiographic contrast medium containing iodine. Iodine, having a high atomic number (53), provides vivid radiopacity to the contrast medium. The latter, being water soluble, need not be removed from the joint following the procedure but is absorbed through the synovium into the blood stream and removed from the body via the kidneys. Although it is theoretically possible to provide soft tissue contrast by making the joint spaces increasingly *radiolucent* by the injection of air or nitrogen, I know of no reports of this technique used in the TMJ. There is a report by *Arnaudow*[2] in which double-contrast TMJ arthrography has been performed using opaque contrast medium and air, though it does not appear to offer significant advantages over purely opaque arthrography.

The goal of TMJ arthrography is to radiographically discern the soft tissue components of the joint. Specifically, we attempt to determine the precise antero-posterior (AP) position of the articular disc and its posterior attachment. In addition, information is sought concerning the morphology of the disc itself and the thickness of the posterior attachment. Thus, the procedure is primarily designed to visualize the soft tissues as a radiolucent void between two opaque pools of contrast medium. Describing the morphology of the joint spaces is only of secondary consideration.

The forms and sizes of the normal upper and

lower joint spaces can be appreciated from a radiograph of a decalcified TMJ, obtained at autopsy from a young adult (Fig. 1). In this illustration, the joint soft tissues are seen at a radiographic density comparable to the decalcified hard tissues. Between the bony surfaces, the biconcave articular disc intervenes, filling virtually the entire interbony space. Curvilinear slivers of the upper and lower joint spaces are seen as relative radiolucencies just covering the bony surfaces. The relatively thick posterior attachment of the disc fills virtually the entire superior and posterior parts of the interbony space. Although the precise junction between the posterior attachment and the disc cannot be seen radiographically, gross and histologic necropsy studies have demonstrated (*Solberg* and *Hansson*[7]) that this junction is at the point indicated by the arrow. Figure 2 illustrates a gross dissection of a fresh autopsy joint specimen, indicating the basic relationship between the disc, the joint spaces, and the articulating bones.

## Pioneers in TMJ arthrography

The first important publication on the subject of TMJ arthrography was *Norgaard's* 1947 monograph[5] entitled "Temporomandibular Arthrography." Many of the important technical concepts that are still employed today have their origin in the work of this earliest pioneer. To quote his preliminary 1944 study[4] of the subject, "I have been working on a method for contrast examination of the joint, and it has yielded some valuable diagnostic information in lesions localized to the nonosseous parts of the joint in a fairly large number of patients without causing more than moderate and transitory inconvenience." In the early 1970's, two significant publications were produced by *Agerberg* and *Lundberg*[1] and by *Toller*[8]. The former authors noted that arthrography provides a valuable aid in the diagnosis of interarticular soft tissue damage. *Toller*, on the other hand, felt that the usefulness of arthrography in clinical research must be contrasted with its limitations in providing clinical diagnoses. Though *Toller* had a guarded appraisal of the procedure for routine clinical work, he gave a detailed description of a workable technique and made important observations on TMJ locking difficulties. In 19 cases of clicking joints studied by arthrography, *Toller* noted that in no case did the condyle ride over the posterior ridge of the meniscus. "Most cases involved a hesitation of the meniscal glide in the upper joint cavity at the point of clicking."

Recently, *Wilkes*[9, 10] published a significant discussion of TMJ arthrographic diagnosis of the TMJ Pain Dysfunction Syndrome. This author carefully correlated clinical features of the syndrome in 400 cases having TMJ arthrography, a large number of which were subsequently operated and inspected visually. *Wilkes* has provided interpretations of the normal TMJ arthrogram and the abnormal presentation found in patients demonstrating painful limitation of opening, clicking, and locking. *Wilkes* has, in the process, upgraded the technical aspects of the examination by prescribing fluoroscopic monitoring of the joint catheter placement procedure and tomographic imaging of the opacified spaces.

## Technical difficulties associated with TMJ arthrography

Despite the successes of the aforementioned individuals, TMJ arthrography remains a technically difficult examination to perform. There are three reasons for this. First, the joint spaces are relatively small.

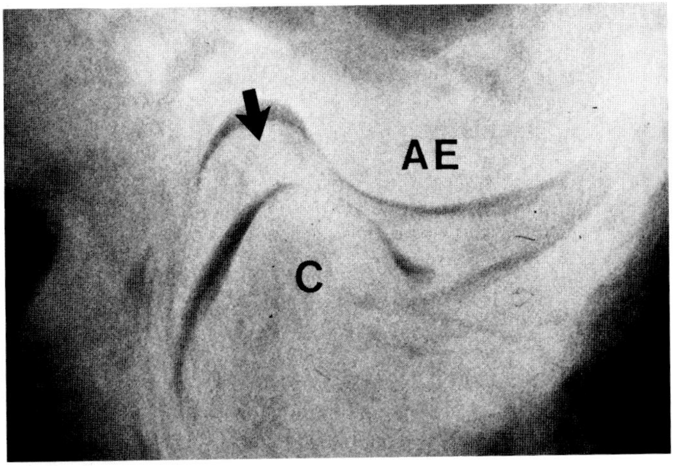


Fig. 1 Decalcified human TMJ obtained at necropsy. The condylar head (C) is seen in apposition to the posterior slope of the articular eminence (AE). Intervening between the bony structures is the articular disc and the posterior attachment. The arrow indicates the approximate junction of the disc and the posterior attachment. The picture is similar to a TMJ arthrogram except that the joint spaces are seen here as radiolucencies. (Necropsy specimen courtesy of Drs. *Tore Hansson* and *William K. Solberg*).

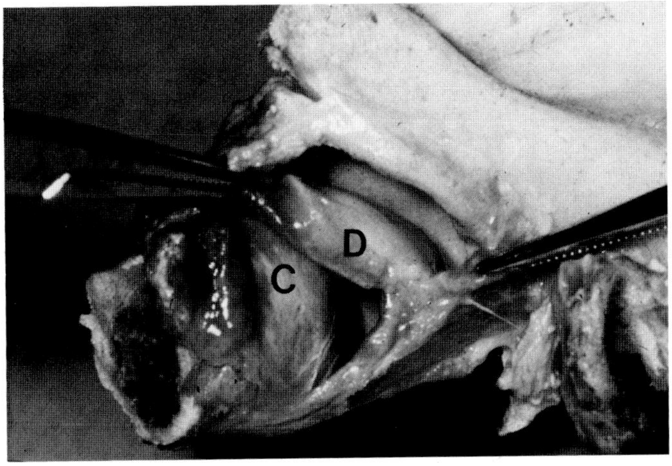


Fig. 2 A gross dissection of a human temporomandibular joint obtained at necropsy shown in lateral presentation. The condylar head (C) has been forcefully distracted from the articular fossa, allowing visualization of the articular disc (D) and the upper and lower joint spaces. (Photograph courtesy of Drs. *Tore Hansson* and *William K. Solberg*).

Needle placement into (or catheterization of) these joint spaces continues to be the most difficult single aspect of the entire examination. Fluoroscopic monitoring helps in this regard but the procedure still requires considerable knowledge of joint anatomy along with skill and experience in the placement of catheters. Secondly, in contrast to the more commonly performed procedure in the knee, TMJ arthrography requires opacification of **two** separate joint spaces for maximum diagnostic information. Though single opacification of the lower space only may provide important information, double joint space opacification is needed to make critical judgments on the position and morphology of the disc (e. g., compression and folding deformations) and on the thickness of the posterior attachment. Finally, assuming one obtains ideal catheterization and infusion of the joint spaces, one is still confronted with traditional difficulties in obtaining clear, nondistorted radiographs of the temporomandibular joint. Whether transcranial radiography or tomography is employed, radiographic technical expertise is more in demand for this small joint than for the analogous procedure performed in the knee.

## Indication and contra-indications

The indication for TMJ arthrography should be made clear before we discuss the interpretation of the examination. At our institution, the sole indication is clinical evidence and/or patient history suggesting internal derangement of the joint soft tissues, including the symptoms classically described by *Schwartz*[6] and *Laskin*[3] indicating TMJ or Myofascial Pain Dysfunction Syndrome. Specifically, these symptoms include pain in the TMJ, painful limitation of opening, deviation of the mandible toward the side of involvement, clicking or popping noises and sporadic or constant locking of the jaw in the partially closed or open positions. A history of progress from clicking to locking is particularly suggestive of serious internal derangement. TMJ arthrography provides its most valuable and needed diagnostic contribution in those cases in which prior TMJ radiographs disclose little or no bony alteration. It is rarely necessary to perform the procedure in cases of severe arthrosis.

Contra-indications include, foremost, allergy or hypersensitivity to the radiographic contrast medium or to iodine itself. All candidates for this procedure are questioned carefully about possible allergic reactions during prior radiological procedures employing an iodinated contrast medium. The procedure should not be performed in cases in which there has been a previous positive allergic reaction. Another contra-indication is articular or para-articular infection, including regional acute infections such as otitis media and parotid gland infection. If such a condition is present, the TMJ arthrogram should be delayed until the infection is definitely controlled. This will prevent the possibility of spreading the infec-
prevent the possibility of spreading the infection in the process of catherizing through it.

## The normal arthrogram

At this juncture, we will turn to the arthrographic appearance of the normal temporomandibular joint. The first illustration in this section (Fig. 3) is derived from a drawing by *Wilkes*[9]. Four stages of joint function are illustrated, from the closed (centric occlusion) position to maximal opening (three fingerbreadths interincisal distance). The white areas between the bony components represent the opacified upper and lower joint spaces, both of which have posterior and anterior recesses. It should be understood that the *filled* joint spaces are artificially distended to some extent by reason of their containing contrast fluid. In the normal, physiologic state, the upper and lower spaces are only *potential* spaces. Notice also that the thin central portion of the articular disc remains between the articulating bony surfaces during all the stages of condyle translation. The thickened posterior portion or rim of the disc always remains slightly posterior to the articulating portion of the condylar head in normal joint function. At full opening, it is seen that the condyle and disc obliterate the lower and upper anterior recesses as contrast medium is hydraulically forced into the posterior recesses.

Actual arthrographic demonstration of the normal condition is provided in a case (Fig. 4) of *Wilkes*, used with his generous permission. In Figures 4a and 4b, upper and lower spaces are opacified in two stages of jaw opening: mild (1 fingerbreadth) opening and full (3 fingerbreadths) jaw opening. No-

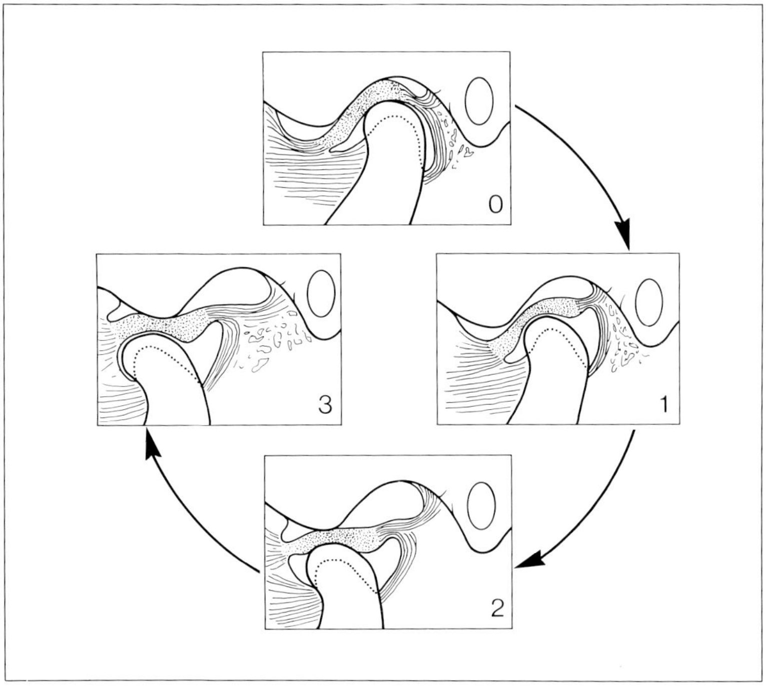


Fig. 3 The normal TMJ hard and soft tissue articulating relationship during opening movement. The four drawings represent the relationships of the disc to bony structures at closed position and various stages of opening, as seen arthrographically. Top, in the closed position (O), the disc is seen as a stippled soft tissue structure between the anterior aspect of the condylar head and the posterior slope of the articular eminence. At one, two and three fingerbreadths opening (1), (2), (3), notice that the thin central portion of the disc maintains the same relationship between the bony surfaces. During jaw opening, the anterior joint space recesses are progressively obliterated while the posterior recesses become larger, assuming shapes that are now recognized as normal. At full opening the posterior recess of the upper space resembles a "D" lying down while the posterior recess of the lower space assumes a "half of a heart" shape. (after *Wilkes, Clyde H.*: Arthrography of the Temporomandibular Joint, *Minnesota Medicine*, November, 1978, Figure 4, used with permission).

tice in the latter that the contrast medium has been forced completely out of the anterior recesses and assumes characteristic shapes as the posterior recesses fill. The contrast medium remains well confined to the two joint spaces, with no evidence of dispersion or spreading into the extracapsular tissues.

## The abnormal arthrogram: the clicking phenomenon

An artist's representation of an arthrogram showing the clicking phenomenon, as modified after *Wilkes*, is seen in Figure 5. A fundamentally important observation is seen in the very top drawing, which indicates the closed

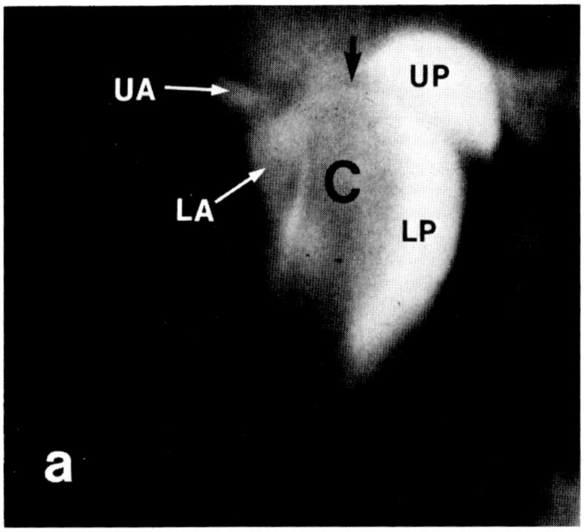


Fig. 4 Normal temporomandibular joint arthrogram.

a) Tomogram of the TMJ following opacification of the upper and lower joint spaces. The patient is at approximately 1 fingerbreadth interincisal opening. Notice the radiographic contrast medium in the upper space, anterior recess (UA); lower space, anterior recess (LA); lower space, posterior recess, (LP); and upper space, posterior recess (UP). The joint spaces are separated by the radiolucency of the articular disc and the posterior attachment. The black arrow indicates the approximate point of junction of disc and posterior attachment.

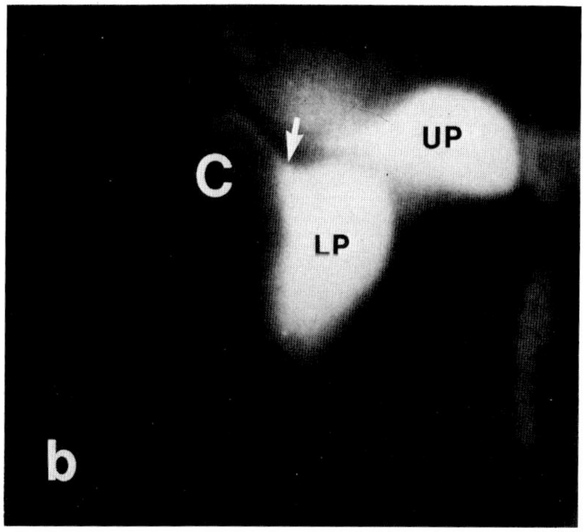


b) Same joint shown at maximal (3 fingerbreadths) jaw opening. The condyle (C) has translated normally to a point anterior to the articular eminence. Notice that there is complete obliteration of the anterior recesses of both joint spaces. There is consequent filling of the posterior recesses (UP and LP). The posterior aspect of the disc (arrow) remains slightly posterior to the articulating surfaces of the bony components. (Figs. 4 a, b, courtesy of *Wilkes, Clyde H.*, Arthrography of the Temporomandibular Joint, *Minnesota Medicine*, November, 1978, Figure 3, used with permission).

jaw joint relationship. Notice that the thickened posterior aspect of the disc is positioned *slightly anterior* to the articulating surface of the condyle. This is a fundamentally different presentation than that noted previously in the normal joint (Fig. 3). During opening translatory movement, the condyle must negotiate the thick "bump," which is the posterior rim of the disc. As the condyle pops under this thickened rim there is often an audible click and a visual "jump" of the disc seen on the fluoroscopic screen. Following this "equilibration" of the disc-condyle relationship, the arthrogram is normal throughout the remaining opening sequence. A case demonstrating this phenomenon is shown in Figure 6. The radiolucent disc between the two pools of contrast is seen to be slightly anterior to the condylar head (Fig. 6a). Specifically, the thickened posterior portion of the disc (arrow) is anterior to the articulating surface (*) of the condylar head. At one fingerbreadth opening (Fig. 6b), the condylar head has passed beneath the thickened posterior rim of the disc and the relationship between soft and hard

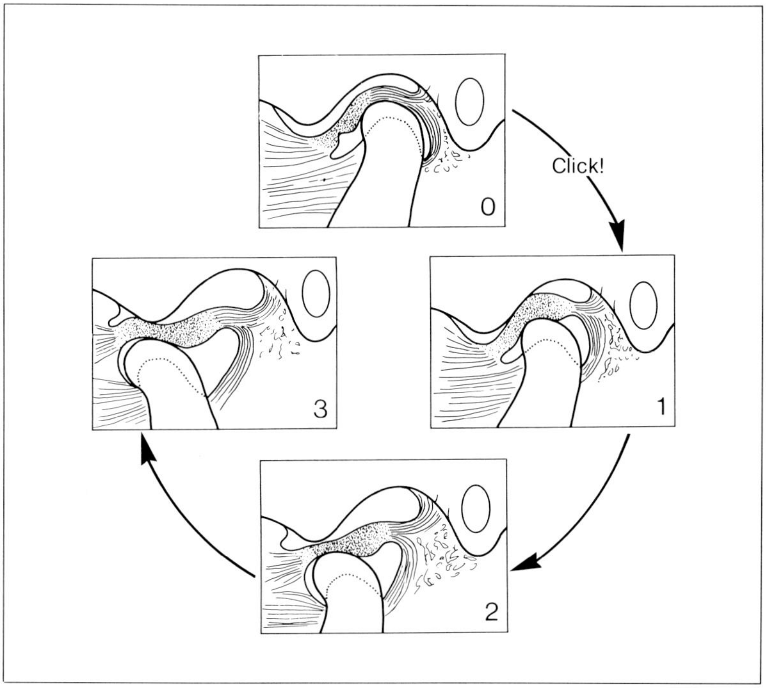


Fig. 5 Internal TMJ derangement--the early click. Notice in the closed position (O) that the biconcave disc (stippled) is situated completely anterior to the articulating surface of the condyle. As the condyle begins to translate anteriorly it passes beneath the thickened rim of the disc at the same time as the patient notices a click within the joint. At one finger-breadth opening (1) and throughout the remaining opening sequence the relationship between disc and bony structures is normal, with articulation taking place through the thin central portion of the disc. (After *Wilkes, Clyde H.*, Arthrography of the Temporomandibular Joint, *Minnesota Medicine*, November, 1978, Figure 8, used with permission).

tissues becomes harmonious for the remaining opening sequence. From this point on, the articulating surfaces of the bones approximate the thin central portion of the disc and the anterior recesses are substantially evacuated of contrast medium.

## The abnormal arthrogram: the locking phenomenon

A more serious clinical presentation occurs when a patient presents with partial or persistent locking of the condyle in an open or closed position. In this section, there will be three demonstrations of such cases in which arthrograms have assisted in the diagnosis of internal derangement of the joint soft tissues. In the last two cases, the arthrographic interpretations were corroborated by the direct inspection of the joints in the process of performing surgical corrections. It would be helpful to first examine a graphic illustration of a hypothetical case representative of the closed locking phenomenon. In Figure 7, the drawings depict alterations in disc form and

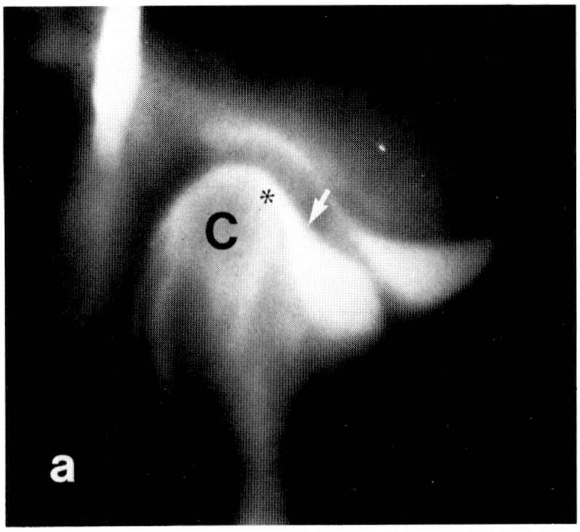


Fig. 6 Arthrogram of joint derangement manifested clinically as an early click.

a) With patient biting in centric occlusion, the condyle (C) is seated in the articular fossa. Upper and lower joint spaces are opacified, especially the anterior recesses, allowing visualiziation of disc and posterior attachment. The main focus of condyle articulation is indicated by.* The articular disc is situated anterior to this point, the arrow denoting the posterior thick portion of the disc. This point would normally be situated over and behind the condyle articulation point.*

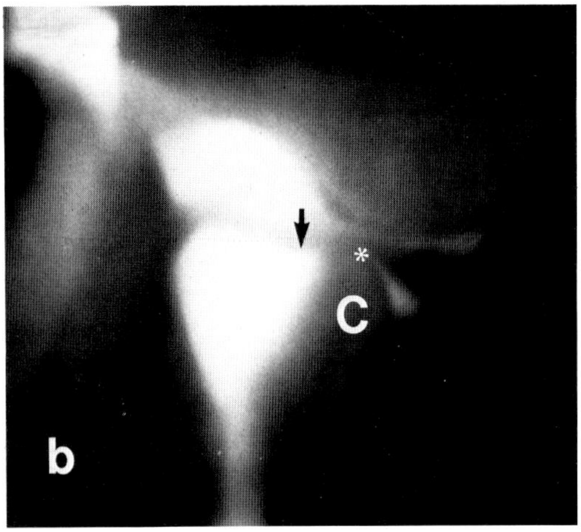


b) At two fingerbreadths opening, the articulating point (*) has passed beneath the thick posterior rim of the articular disc (arrow). At the precise point during which the patient felt and heard a click within the joint, the condylar articulation passed under the posterior aspect of the disc. Notice the normal hydraulic movement of contrast away from the anterior recesses.

position which have been shown to occur both in *Wilkes'* material[9, 10] and in numerous cases evaluated at the UCLA School of Dentistry. The top drawing, Figure 7a, is essentially identical to Figure 5a, showing that the posterior aspect of the disc is situated anterior to the condylar head with the teeth in occlusion, the only difference being that in Figure 7a the disc is so altered in morphology that it has lost its biconcavity. The disc appears as an amorphous, deformed mass of soft tissue. During opening translatory movement, the condyle is not able to negotiate or ride under the thickened mass of the disc but, rather, mechanically forces the disc forward by shearing action (Fig. 7 c). At the locking point, the condylar head is prevented from attaining its normal anterior position by the mechanical obstruction of the displaced disc and possibly also by the maximal stretching of the posterior attachment.

Case number 1 is a 14-year-old girl who presented with a two year history of clicking and painful limitation of opening of the left TMJ. Figures 8 a and 8 b are arthrograms in closed and slightly opened jaw positions. The disc

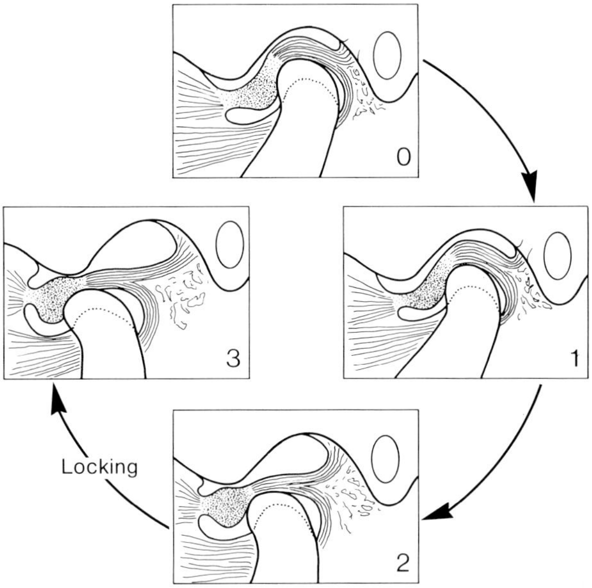


Fig. 7 Severe disc derangement—the closed lock situation. In the closed projection at the top (0 fingerbreadths interincisal opening) notice that the stippled disc has been deformed from normal biconcave wafer to an amorphous mass. The disc is situated entirely anterior to the condylar articulating surface. During stages of jaw opening, the condyle progressively forces the disc mass anteriorly, causing greater deformation. At no point in this sequence does the condyle negotiate its way past the thickened posterior aspect of the disc to acquire a normal relationship. As the disc is compressed forward there is a consequent stretching of the posterior attachment.

(D) is clearly abnormally forward of the condyle (C) in these two pictures. Figure 8c represents the maximum open position that the patient could attain. Several key diagnostic findings are evident: First, the anterior recesses of the upper and lower spaces are not obliterated (i. e., by evacuation of contrast medium) as they should be in the normal condition. Secondly, the disc is seen as a radiolucent mass situated anterior to the partially translated condylar head. The displaced disc forms a mechanical obstruction to anterior movement of the condyle. Figure 8d is a line drawing representing this situation.

Case number 2 is that of a 26-year-old woman who had an eight year history of intermittent closed locking of right condylar movement, associated with pain on opening. In the early stages, the patient noticed intermittent clicking within this joint. Figure 9a is the arthrogram made with both joint spaces opacified, and with the patient at one fingerbreadth jaw opening. As with most arthrograms, precise determination of the condylar position in this case is hindered by the

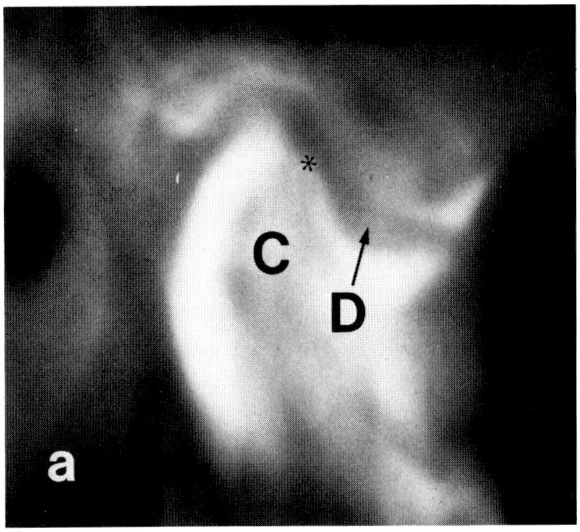


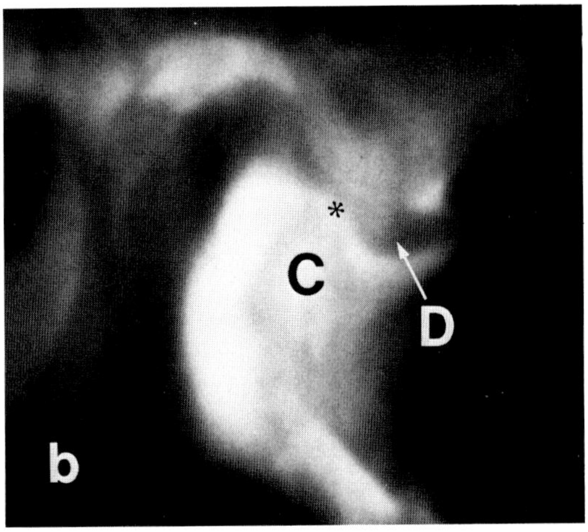


Fig. 8 Case # 1, temporomandibular joint locking.

a) The arthrogram shows the disc (D) as a radiolucency between the anterior recesses. The disc is displaced anterior to the primary focus of condylar articulation (*). The patient is at one fingerbreadth interincisal opening.

b) At 2 fingerbreadths, the disc remains displaced. The disc becomes further deformed while the anterior recesses retain abnormally large volumes of contrast.

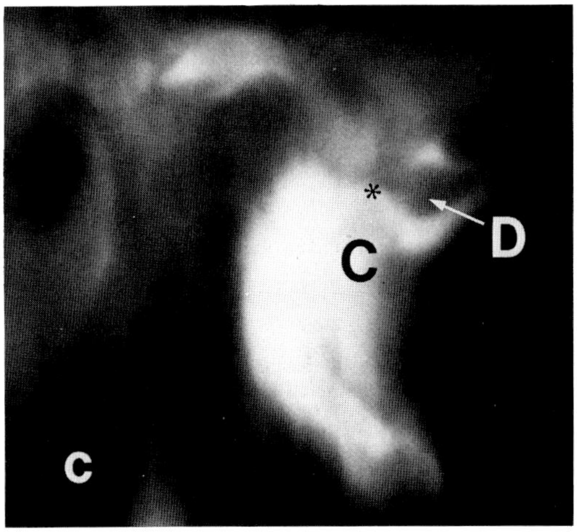


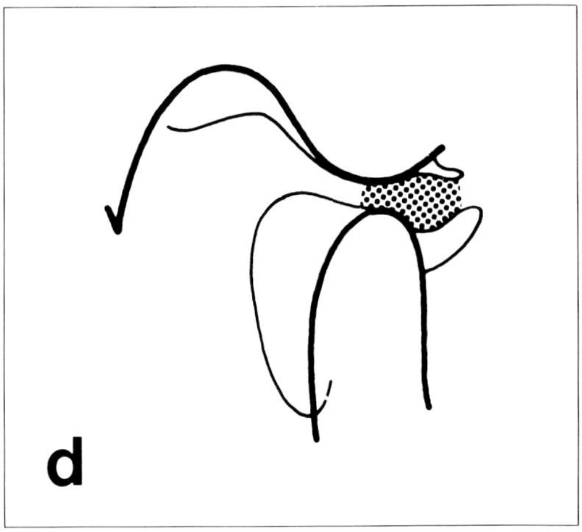


c) At maximal opening, the disc has been forced further anteriorly, retaining its displaced relationship with the condylar head. The anterior recesses retain contrast medium because the disc forms a mechanical obstruction.

d) A graphic representation of (c) is shown. The disc is seen as the stippled area. The disc, instead of showing the normal biconcave shape, is deformed.

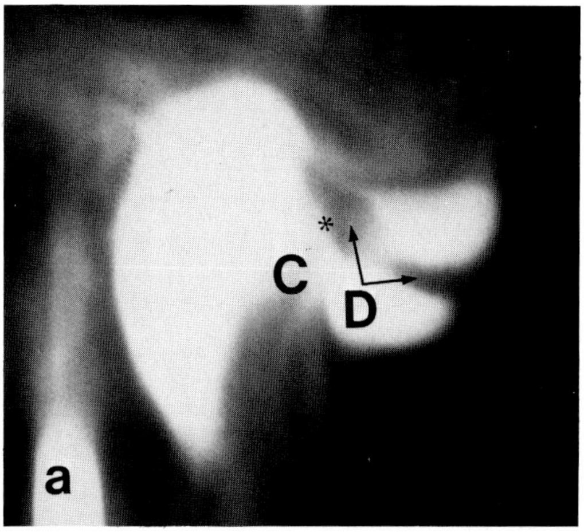


Fig. 9 Case # 2, TMJ disc derangement manifested by closed lock.

a) The biconcave shaped disc is denoted by arrows pointing to the relatively thick anterior and posterior portions. Again, the entire disc is positioned anterior to the condylar head (C); specifically, the articulating point of the condylar head (*). (The posterior attachment to the disc and the thin central portion of the disc are obliterated by the densely opaque shadows of the joint spaces).

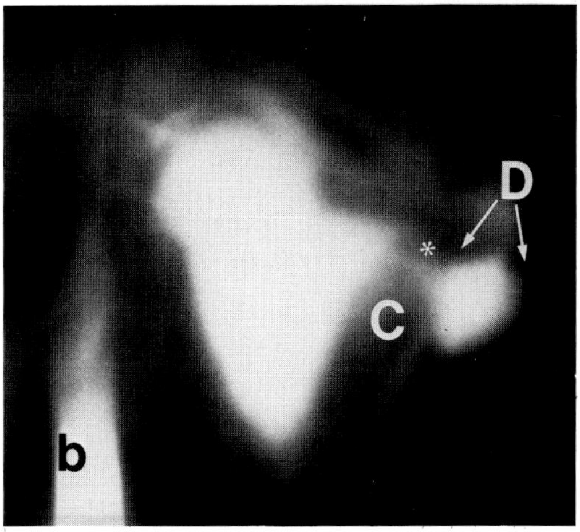


b) The maximal opening situation is represented. The condyle (C) has forced the disc (D) severely forward in the joint. The disc forms a mechanical obstruction to further condyle translation; pressure from the condyle has in turn deformed the disc. White arrows point to the short, relatively thickened anterior and posterior aspects of the disc.

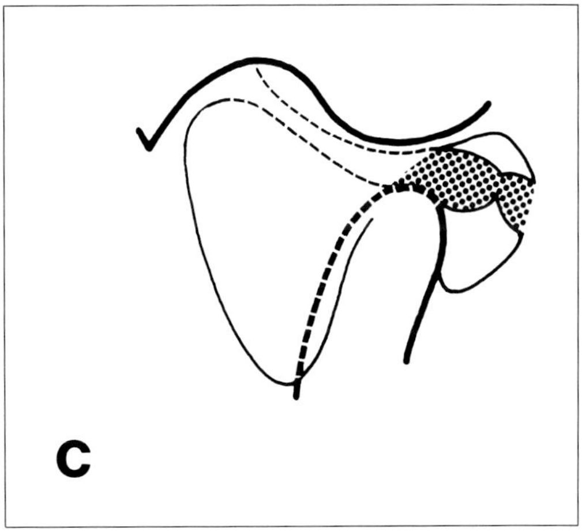


c) Graphic illustration of (b). The compressed mass of the disc is seen as the stippled area anterior to the articulating point of the condylar head. The disc has a deformed, bilobed shape. Notice the residual contrast remaining in the anterior recesses.

contrast medium surrounding the condylar head, but clearly the condylar head (C) is situated somewhat posteriorly to the posterior rim of the disc (arrow). At maximal opening (Fig. 9 b), two cardinal arthrographic features of the closed lock are apparent: 1) the anterior joint space recesses retain contrast medium, a fact that reflects the inability of the condyle to fully translate anteriorly; and 2) the radiolucent shadow of the disc remains clearly anterior to the articulating portion of the condylar head, indicating that the cause of the limitation is obstruction by the disc itself. The deformation of the disc is seen more clearly in line drawing form in Figure 9 c.

Case numbers 3 is that of a 20-year-old man who sustained a traumatic blow to the jaw during a football scrimmage two years prior to the arthrogram. During the two year interval, the patient experienced chronic closed lock of the right condyle during opening jaw movements, pain upon opening and, until one year previously, clicking within this joint. The arthrogram (Fig. 10a, b), illustrates derangement in the slightly open and maximal open jaw relationships. The posterior thick portion of the disc (D) is seen to be anterior to the condyle (C) with the patient's mouth slightly open. At maximal opening (Fig. 10b), the contrast medium has been evacuated from the anterior recess of the upper space, though a considerable amount remains in the anterior recess of the lower space. The conformation of the visualized anterior recess of the lower space is highly specific and demonstrates what I like to call the "spike sign" (between the arrows). The opaque spike, pointing superiorly, indicates a crease in the disc which is folded like a wallet about its central portion. This is seen graphically in Figure 10c. The disc appears to form a physical obstruction to maximal condylar translation. The premise in this and similar cases is that the compressive force of the condyle has forced the pliable disc to become folded.

The above arthrograms are made with tomographic images of the opacified joint spaces. Tomograms, however, can only provide images at specific points in time, during which functional and dysfunctional movements of the joint structures take place. For this reason, fluoroscopic visualization was utilized in all of these cases in order to provide continuous interpretation of joint movements. Fluoroscopy is recommended to give the operator complimentary findings and clarification on the position and the behavior of the disc during specific phases of joint clicking and locking.

## TMJ arthrographic technique

The arthrographic technique I use is a modification of *Wilkes'*. It has proven to be consistently successful, without major postarthrographic pain and discomfort for the patient. In this section emphasis will be placed on the most important technical aspects that should be observed in performing this procedure. To begin, it is best to perform the procedure in a medical radiology department or office since specialized radiographic equipment is required. It is of considerable technical advantage to perform the procedure in a room having both fluoroscopic and tomographic capabilities. In addition, it is helpful to recline the patient so that the head is supported by a firm surface, such as a table top, to facilitate joint space catheterization.

Strict aseptic technique must be observed in the performance of the examination. With the patient lying on the radiology table, and with the side of interest up, the preauricular area is thoroughly cleansed with a disinfecting solution and isolated with a sterile drape. Local anesthesia of the preauricular soft tis-

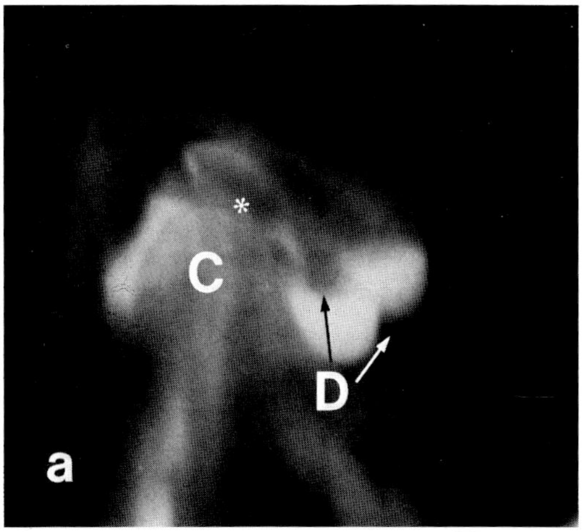


Fig. 10 Case # 3, disc obstruction of condyle translation shown as the "spike sign."

a) The condyle (C) is moderately well-seated in the articular fossa. The anterior and posterior portions of the disc (D) are denoted by white and black arrows. (The thin central portion of the disc is obliterated by contrast superimposition). The articulating point of the condylar head (*) is seen against the posterior attachment.

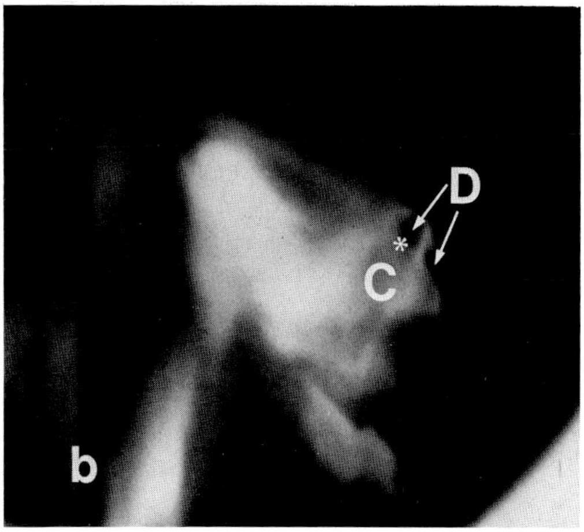


b) At maximal opening the shadow of the condyle is not clearly seen but is judged to be in the approximate position of (C). The condyle has forced the disc to fold like a wallet, trapping a small column of contrast medium between the two arms of the disc (arrows). The "spike sign" is seen as the slender column of opaque substance between the two arrows.

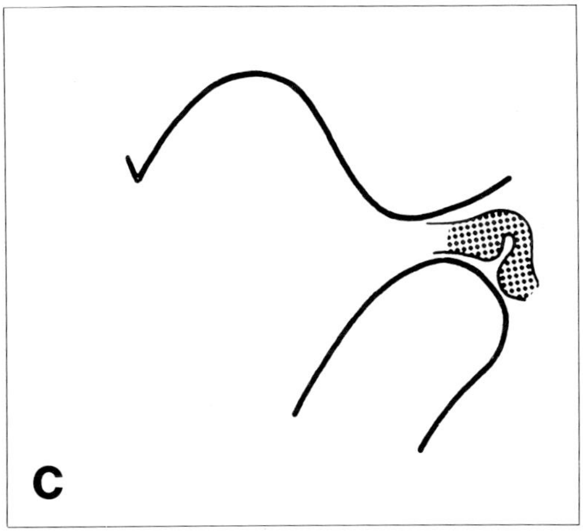


c) Graphic illustration. The disc is seen as the stippled structure having thickened anterior and posterior portions folded around the thin central portion. Contrast in the lower space is clearly seen as the "spike" reaching into the bifurcation of the disc.

sues and the para-articular structures is obtained by injection of lidocaine 1% with 1 : 100,000 concentration of epinephrine (Fig. 12a). A small amount of local anesthetic solution is injected into the joint space, providing positive intra-articular fluid pressure.

The process of catheterizing the joint spaces begins, and the patient is asked to open his mouth moderately. A catheter-needle combination (20 or 22 gauge angiocatheter) is inserted into the tissue in the direction of the posterior recess of the lower space (Fig. 12b). Positive intra-articular placement of the angiocatheter tip may be assured by 1) observing the placement fluoroscopically while palpating the posterior surface of the condylar head with the catheter tip and by 2) the ability to easily inject the fluid. The syringe-needle combination is withdrawn, *leaving in place* the flexible outer catheter. At this point, the patient is asked to close his mouth and a slight regurgitation of excess local anesthetic from the hub of the catheter will signify that the catheter is, indeed, placed within the joint space.

A different syringe, containing water-soluble contrast medium, attached to a stopcock and flexible plastic tubing, is connected to the hub of the angio-catheter (Fig. 12 c). Care must be taken to assure that no air bubbles exist in the line before making this connection. (During this time, the patient's eyeblink reflex should be checked periodically to assure that it has not been partially blocked by the local anesthetic. If the eyeblink reflex is overly sluggish, it is recommended that the eyelid be taped closed to prevent foreign matter from lodging in the cornea). Figure 12d shows the examination site following catheterization of both upper and lower spaces and connections to the syringes containing contrast medium.

At this point, preliminary (scout) tomograms are made of the joint in order to assure that correct exposure factors and focal cuts are used on subsequent "opacified" tomograms. When the technical factors are optimally set, lower space opacification may begin. Injection of very slight amounts of contrast medium should be performed under fluoroscopic monitoring to insure that an intra-articular injection is being made. Also during this time, the operator should determine that the contrast medium is flowing into the lower joint space only. If there is concurrent opacification of the upper joint space, one has positive indication of a pathologic connection between the two spaces through a rent or perforation of the disc. If no perforation is shown, the operator completes filling of the lower space to a maximum of 0.7 cc or until he feels positive back pressure on the syringe plunger. Tomograms are made in closed and graded opening jaw relationships.

The operator immediately fills the upper joint space with a maximum of 0.8 cc of contrast medium, or again until positive back pressure is felt, all the time monitoring the upper space filling fluoroscopically. Tomograms are again made with the jaws closed and with the joint in various stages of function. Only at this point are the radiographs inspected. Filling both joint spaces prior to examination of the tomograms insures that the tomography process is performed expediently and without delay. It is critically important to avoid a time delay before tomographic images are made, as water-soluble contrast medium begins to disperse into the synovium and vascular spaces of the posterior attachment within 10 to 15 minutes following injection. This dispersion of contrast medium increasingly blurs the outlines of the disc and posterior attachment. Detailed fluoroscopic and tomographic visualization must be obtained quickly after opacification.

If the tomograms are found to be adequate, the examination can be terminated as

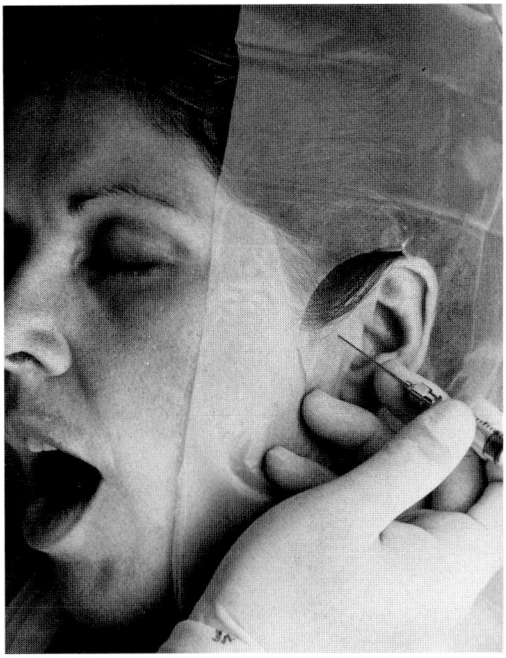

Fig. 11 TMJ arthrographic technique.

a) In anesthetizing the preauricular soft tissues, the operator is placing a 27 gauge needle in the direction of the upper joint space. The preauricular soft tissues have been scrubbed and isolated with a sterile drape.

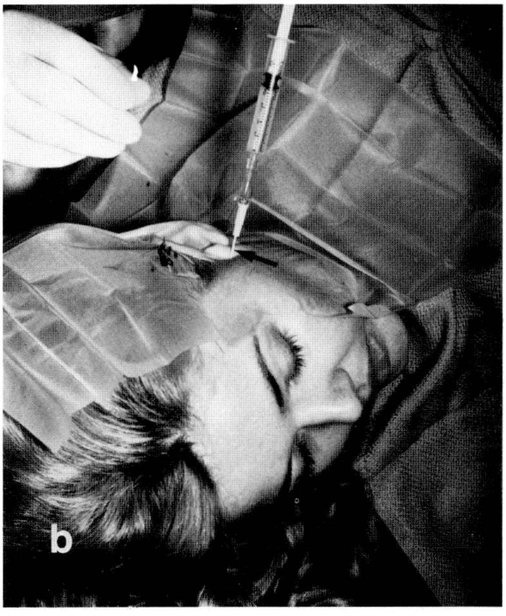


b) Joint space catheterization. The black arrow points to a 22 gauge angiocatheter partially inserted in the soft tissues in the direction of the posterior recess of the lower joint space. The syringe contains 1 % lidocaine solution. The process of gradually inserting the angiocatheter into the tissues is monitored fluoroscopically.

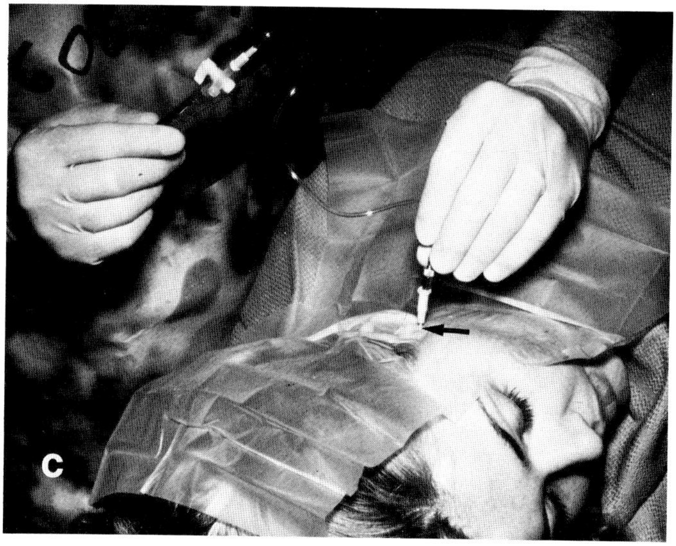

c) When the lower joint space is entered, the central stylet is removed and the outer catheter is advanced slightly. The operator then connects a syringe-stopcock-tube combination to the catheter to form a closed injection system. This illustration shows the operator making the connection between tubing and catheter.

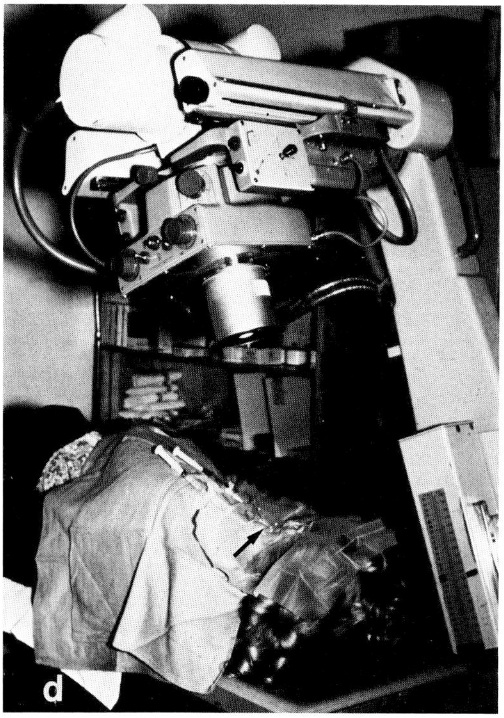

d) The arthrogram site (cranial-posterior aspect). The black arrow is pointing to two angiocatheters which have been placed into the joint spaces. Two syringes containing the radiographic contrast medium are taped to sterile towels. The X-ray tube is oriented in the transcranial position. The X-ray machine can also be programmed to make tomographic projections of the TMJ.

follows: The operator should attempt to aspirate contrast medium from both upper and lower joint spaces, though this action is very often unproductive or only slightly productive. The angiocatheters are removed slowly. They should be inspected to be sure that they are intact. Pressure should be applied to the arthrogram site with sterile gauze, followed by an icepack. Analgesics may be prescribed to ameliorate the patient's expected postarthrographic discomfort. Most patients will experience moderate discomfort, especially upon opening, the night of the arthrogram and with diminishing intensity for several days following the procedure. The patient's dental occlusion on the side of the arthrogram may also be altered, gradually returning to the prearthrogram state within a short period of time.

## Summary

*With regard to the TMJ Arthrographic Procedure:* TMJ arthrography may be performed with fairly consistent technical success, without significant complications, and with only moderate side effects, i. e., discomfort and altered occlusion following the procedure. This outcome presupposes that the arthrographer is thoroughly familiar with TMJ anatomy and function, and that the procedure is performed with aseptic technique in an adequately equipped radiology facility (one having at the very least fluoroscopic and hopefully also tomographic capability). The lower space certainly, and ideally the upper space also, must be adequately filled but not overfilled with water-soluble contrast medium. Finally, the jaw opening radiographs are made expediently and without delay following joint space filling.

*With regard to TMJ Arthrographic Interpretation:* The internal soft tissues of the TMJ, i.e., the disc and its posterior attachment, can be radiographically visualized and a determination can be made of the position and morphology of the disc in various stages of joint function. Positioning of the disc anterior to the condylar head is the most common abnormality seen. Depending on the severity of the disc displacement and deformity, and other unknown factors, the disc may cause a definite obstruction to complete anterior condyle translation (i.e., closed locking). In cases of lesser severity (i.e., clicking), the condyle may pass under the posterior aspect of the disc to assume a more harmonious relationship for the remainder of the translatory movement. These phenomena, as seen on a fluoroscopic screen during arthrography, can be clearly correlated with the clinical presentation of an audible click or a closed lock. It must also be said that TMJ arthrography is still in an early stage of development and it is necessary to have considerable clinical and surgical correlation of normal and abnormal findings in order to produce confident interpretations.

### References

1. *Agerberg, G.,* and *Lundberg, M.*
Changes in the temporomandibular joint after surgical treatment. Oral Surg. 32: 865–875, 1971.
2. *Arnaudow, V. M.:*
Die Doppelkontrast-arthrotomographic des Kiefergelenkes, DZZ 23: 390–393, 1968.
3. *Laskin, D. M.:*
Etiology of the pain-dysfunction syndrome. J. Am. Dent. Assoc. 79: 147–153, 1969.
4. *Norgaard, F.:*
Arthrography of the mandibular joint. Acta Radiol. 25: 679–685, 1944.
5. Idem: Temporomandibular Arthrography. Copenhagen. *Einar Munksgaard,* 1974.
6. *Schwartz, L.:*
The pain-dysfunction syndrome. In Schwartz, L., and Chayes, C. M., Facial Pain and Mandibular Dysfunction, Philadelphia, W. B. Saunders Co., 1968, p. 140–155.

7. *Solberg, W. K.*, and *Hansson, T.*:
Personal communication, 1979.

8. *Toller, P. A.*:
Opaque arthrography of the temporomandibular joint. Int. J. Oral Surg. 3: 17–28, 1974.

9. *Wilkes, Clyde H.*
Arthrography of the Temporomandibular Joint. Minnesota Medicine, November, 1978, p. 645–652.

10. *Wilkes, Clyde H.*:
Structural and functional alterations of the temporomandibular joint. Northwest Dentistry, 57: 287–294, 1978b.

## Discussion

Discussant: Tore Hansson

*Dr. Hansson*

This is my first opportunity to say to the Symposium organization that I am very happy to be here. I will also say to Dr. *Blaschke* that this was a great contribution to the Symposium and to furthering the diagnostic methodology of temporomandibular joint diseases. As Dr. *Moffett* stressed this morning, this technique might help us out of the confusion involving different dysfunctions or at least different aspects of the same phenomena. You know already, Dr. *Blaschke*, that the soft tissue aspects of the TMJ are very close to my heart, and of course I was happy to see your application of arthrography for that purpose. But I would like to comment about the anterior displacement of discs, because I know over here in the United States you see many more anteriorly displaced discs than we do in Sweden, and I'm curious to learn much more about it. I am really looking forward to your developing this technique further so we can argue in a friendly way about it! First of all, what is your opinion about the clinical diagnosis of the problem before you do the radiographic examination? Swedish radiologists are very careful when we send referrals to them. They really want the clinical diagnosis of the problem before they take any radiograms. How do you feel about this in regard to arthrography procedures?

*Dr. Blaschke*

Well, when I have been given a request to do this procedure, it has been my policy to talk personally with the referring clinician. I am not comfortable performing any radiological examination capriciously, of course; especially so with arthrography because we don't really know if there are long-term complications. Everything has been good, so far. I have to understand clearly the history and clinical findings before we schedule a patient. It's not a procedure to do for example simply because a clinician doesn't like the way a condyle lines up with a fossa on a transcranial radiograph.

*Dr. Hansson*

From autopsy material, which is now being investigated at UCLA in the Section of Gnathology and Occlusion, we have seen anteriorly displaced discs, but I would just ask you if the amount and pressure of the contrast medium could possibly have caused the anterior displaced disc?

*Dr. Blaschke*

That is an excellent question, and I have no doubts that the procedure itself artificially affects to some degree what is going on in the joint. One patient I discussed today had an apparently normal arthrogram with just the lower space opacified and then a clearly abnormal arthrogram with both spaces opacified. Even with the small volumes that are injected, one can actually see, fluoroscopically, the posterior attachment moving up and down under the pressures of infusion and aspiration of contrast. One can, therefore, affect the superior-inferior positioning of these tissues as the contrast medium is injected. This is an artifact, of course, but the important consideration is that we don't believe that this or any other arthrography artifact produces anterior disc dislocation. Even if the spaces are overdistended, there is no logical reason to presume that the infusion forces the disc anteriorly. I can't prove it; that is just my feeling.

*Dr. Hansson*

I'm very happy to see the clarity of the soft tissues in your arthrograms. There have been some studies in Sweden by *Omnell* and coworkers (*Nanthaviroj*, 1976) that show there was a bigger interarticular distance before the click than just afterwards, as measured on transcranial radiograms. I was so happy to see that it is exactly in the same region of the joint as your arthrography cases.

*Dr. Blaschke*

I have been able to go back to our prearthrographic tomograms and evaluate joint bony relationships. It is true that there is an increased space between the two bone surfaces before a click, and we are indebted to Dr. *Omnell* for this. We can see other subtle changes on the prearthrographic films. Dr. *William Farrar*, I think, had one of the first articles in 1972, in which he showed that disc derangement anteriorly is usually associated with posterior positioned condyles. I can assure you that many of these positive arthrograms have revealed, on retrospective analysis, that the condyle was retruded within the mandibular fossa, probably to accommodate the disc in front of it. Good point!

*Dr. Solberg*

Are there any comments from the speakers' table? . . . Dr. *Mahan.*

*Dr. Mahan*

One of the things it would be interesting to know, Dr. *Blaschke,* is what's happening when that fluid is not in there? We can't have a vacuum in the tissues, and there is practically no synovial fluid there prior to the injection. I am thinking that, for example, when the condyle comes forward and those recesses fill, that the capsule may be pulled into the area and the blood vessels expand in the vascular knee part, so you would temporarily have a lot thicker meniscus in that region. Do you have any ideas regarding this?

*Dr. Blaschke*

Well, that's a reasonable observation. As Dr. *Mahan* said this morning, TM joint spaces are not aspirable. I routinely attempt to aspirate at the early stage of arthrography but I can't get any fluid back, unlike knee arthrography, and so I feel that these are indeed potential spaces. The engorgement of the venous sinuses posteriorly and possibly the alterations of the capsular form can help modify those spaces as the condyle is coming forward. Arthrographically, I guess we are distorting those spaces by the injection of fluid.

*Dr. Mahan*

Isn't it true in your cases that the injection of the contrast medium doesn't really change the clicking and the other symptoms much?

*Dr. Blaschke*

Yes, that is true. I question patients thoroughly beforehand, and watch them go through clicking maneuvers. Even before I inject the contrast, I observe the opening movements many times on the fluoroscope. It is easy to observe the clicking prior to and during arthrography and it doesn't seem to change, at least in my experience, with regard to the precise point of the click. Maybe *Bill McCarty* has more to give us on that tomorrow.

*Dr. Laskin*

Could the presence of the catheters within the joint spaces have any influence on the position of the disc?

*Dr. Blaschke*

I don't believe so. It is a consideration that has occurred to me. These are really very small catheters, either 20 or 22 gauge, and they are Teflon and therefore quite flexible. They conform to the changes in shape of the fossa, because as the fossa curves over, the catheters can follow the curve. Your question is a theoretical consideration and it is as yet an unknown. I think, however, that for the valuable information that we receive from arthrography, it is worthwhile to go ahead and do them, even though one cannot disprove that the catheters produce an effect on disc position.

*Dr. Solberg*

Dr. *Öberg*, do you have any comment on the disc's ability to dislocate?

*Dr. Öberg*

Dr. *Blaschke*, do you think there are some ruptures in the posterior attachment of the disc when they are dislocated so much? As Dr. *Mahan* has told us earlier, the disc is attached very firmly to the condyle, and I think it functions normally by rotating.

*Dr. Blaschke*

Are you asking for my interpretation of the mechanism that allows an anterior dislocation? Basically, I subscribe to the viewpoints of *Bill Solberg* and *Clyde Wilkes*, as I think many others here do, that there is stretching or a tearing of the posterior attachment which allows the disc to be pushed forward. *Wilkes* has seen this effect surgically, and we have had corroboration according to Dr. *Bruce Sanders* at UCLA, the condyle is positioned in a hernia sac instead of articulating normally below the disc. In severe derangement cases the condyle appears to articulate on the posterior attachment. Over a long period of time the condyle stretches it and a little sac tends to form in there.

*Dr. Farhood* (Santa Maria, California)

A brief comment. I have noticed that an anteriorly displaced disc has a great deal of flab: it is flabby, it is atonic, with no fluid in either of the compartments. The disc dislocates readily when you manipulate the mandible. I was trained in San Antonio with Dr. *Frank Dolwick*. We have done many arthrograms there, and we had a rule of thumb observation that those patients who have experienced the greatest amount of post-arthrographic pain seemed to have had the greatest pathology clinically.

*Dr. Blaschke*

I agree that the patients with the most severe clinical problems presenting for arthrography tend to do worse, and sometimes this discomfort can go on for a week or two. When we have an "early click" case or a normal patient, they tend to be less bothered by postarthrographic discomfort. With regard to postarthrographic pain in general, to some extent it may not just be a result of distention of the joint spaces, but actually a reaction to the iodinated contrast material. I do know that if you inject this iodinated contrast subcutaneously it burns; it conceivably could irritate the joint synovium to some extent.

*Dr. Laskin*

Do you ever find patients where clinically you have made a diagnosis of internal derangement, and you get a normal arthrogram?

*Dr. Blaschke*

Yes. I won't say a normal arthrogram, but a couple of times I have been very surprised at how mild a particular clinical problem looked arthrographically. I am thinking of one particular case I showed here as an "early click." That fellow had a closed lock clinically and painful limitation of opening. When I consulted his surgeon about the arthrography, he just couldn't understand the mildness of the arthrogram in view of the seriousness of the clinical situation. Clearly, there is more to TMJ arthrogram interpretation than I am now aware of.

*Dr. Donald Jones* (New Jersey)

I was wondering if we could poll the speakers this afternoon concerning the etiology of the click, because this latest explanation is contrary to my original understanding that the condyle would ride up the anterior border of the disc and then the disc would catch up.

*Dr. Blaschke*

I try to make sense of the arthrograms based on what clinicians such as Dr. *Solberg* and Dr. *Öberg* tell me from a more basic standpoint. I can't help but feel when I look at these arthrograms that there is a shearing force of that condyle against that enlarged posterior lip of the disc such that it actually forces that disc forward. I really believe that if the disc were normally positioned over the head of the condyle, that wouldn't happen. Now whether it is laxity in the posterior attachment elastic fibers or incoordination of muscles, or irregularities on the articular surfaces which cause that, I can't say.

*Dr. Solberg*

Any comments from the speakers table?

*Dr. Mahan*

Let me say that *Toller*, for example, interpreted his radiographs as though the meniscus were hesitating. The condyle begins to move out, leaving the meniscus behind as it sticks; then, at a given point, it catches up. Our observations have been that when we are palpating the condyle, and the patient opens, at the time of the click we feel tissue move back against our finger. What we had interpreted that to mean was that the meniscus was actually slipping over the back of the condyle. Here we were assuming that at the beginning of the movement the condyle is seated in the pocket and not anteriorly displaced. When we felt the tissue flick back against the finger, we were assuming that the meniscus is slipping posteriorly as the condyle is going over the anterior lip. However, if the condyle is one notch posterior at the outset, with the meniscus entirely in front of the condyle, as the condyle moves it could slip forward onto the disc. But either way, our clinical evidence of feeling the tissue move back against our finger is going to be the same, and the starting point is what makes the difference.

*Dr. Solberg*

Let's have a comment by Dr. *Hansson.*

*Dr. Hansson*

I would just give you another opinion. Based on epidemiological data together with microscopic necropsy data, we have about the same percentage of clicking and crepitation in standardized and representative samples of the population in Scandinavia, as we have found from the autopsy studies which have been performed in Scandinavia and here, in Los Angeles. I think I confess to the theory that local injuries, remodeling of the soft tissue of the articulating layers, and local secondary injuries on the disc are also capable of creating clicking and crepitation.

*Dr. Carl Rieder* (Newport Beach, California)

Dr. *Solberg*, I would like to ask a question on behalf of, I think, a lot of people here. That is, with the epidemiological studies for average adult Americans, and I am sure this bears out in Scandinavia as well, probably a third of clinically normal patients exhibit some type of clicking. Now for us out here in private practice, who find that one-third of our patients exhibit a click, how would you direct us based on this information and on the assumption of a progressive aggravation of this condition? How would you direct us to consider the treatment and when should that treatment be instigated?

*Dr. Solberg*

I will refer this question back to the table . . .

*Dr. Krogh-Poulsen*

Well, I would like to comment, because I think that a click is several things. I think there may be three or four different conditions which make the same symptom. It may be that the disc is held back in one way or the other by a change in the bilaminar zone; in that case I think we will get a click when the condyle passes by the anterior part of the disc in the wide opening—the terminal click. Another thing is that which has been described now [anterior displaced disc]. But a third condition has not yet been mentioned and that is the incoordination of the activity of the upper and lower part of the lateral pterygoid muscle. I think that this plays a role in some kinds of clicks. One time I had the opportunity to examine a patient who had a click in the right joint. In his history it was revealed that he was one day, in his kitchen, fixing some electricity up in the ceiling, when he fell from the table on which he was standing, and received a blow on his chin. He was taken to the hospital with great pain in the right TMJ, but there was no fracture. Apparently, there was a contusion of the joint. A few weeks later, he was absolutely free of symptoms. Then one month later, the right joint started clicking. This clicking went on and on in intensity, and at last, it was so loud that nobody would eat with him. So, at the surgical department of that school where I was examining him, they were considering extirpation of the disc. I examined him using my usual procedure, which includes contact of the teeth in different positions. As I listened with a stethoscope to the joints, he made contact between the lower right and the upper left central. He would move his mandible a little bit to the left side. I then observed that the incisal edge of that upper central incisor had a chip of the enamel broken off, and that he had developed a habit of moving his mandible to this place and every time when he came to that place, the click would come. Now I thought it could be that there was an incoordination in the activity of the upper and lower part of lateral pterygoid muscle, so I asked his permission just to grind this little place, and after I had ground this off, it was impossible for him to click again. I think he had developed a reflex arc acting at that specific position of the mandible, and thus creating a particular disc-condyle relationship through the incoordination of the activities of the upper and lower heads of the lateral pterygoid muscle. This reflex arc was apparently broken by reshaping of the tooth contact.

# V. The Significance of Occlusion in Temporomandibular Function and Dysfunction

by W. Krogh-Poulsen

I have always been interested in the clinical side of TMJ problems and my opinions and concepts have been formed mainly on the basis of clinical observations through the years. Three observations were found especially impressive, and are worth further consideration. The first is the perfect way in which nature has built the stomatognathic system and its functionally associated structures so that structures and activities (form and function) are in working harmony, not only under normal conditions, but also during minor changes. The second observation is that while minor obstacles in the occlusal contact relationships or in oral habits and behavior may trigger the development of pathological conditions in some patients, even major changes such as loss of many teeth, may cause no pathologic effect in others. The third observation is that general factors, such as personal reactions to situations in daily life, play an important role in the behavior, not only of the person as a whole, but also on the stomatognathic system. My thoughts on these phenomena are background for this lecture.

The World Health Organization points out that health is not merely the absence of disease; health is a state of well-being, not only with respect to the body, but also mentally and socially, i. e. in communication with others: family, friends and co-workers. This gives us a clue to observing and understanding patients with disorders resulting from oro-mandibular dysfunction. The well-being is hampered in these patients; either somatically as in cases of impaired mobility of the mandible or painful chewing, or psychically, as in patients with perpetual pain in the ears or the troat which make them irritable or bring them into a state of anxiety, as in the case of a possible malignancy. A characteristic feature is that in many cases several factors are contributing to the etiology of the disorder or dysfunction. An example: A 13-year-old girl had developed a tension headache from the left temporal muscle, because she had clenched her front teeth edge-to-edge with such force that the enamel at certain places was chipped off. The school dentist observed the irregular incisal attrition, but the patient did not tell about her headaches. She was just in for a routine check-up. The dentist asked her to press her front teeth against each other and stay put. The effect was that the well-known headache very soon was established. But a 13-year-old girl does not get headaches or brux her teeth to such a degree without having a special background. Further talk with the girl showed that the situation at home caused much psychic tension in the patient. In her case, it was a social problem that expressed itself in the bruxism and headaches. This girl was not ill, but her well-being and her welfare were hampered.

The background is multifactorial (Fig. 1). In this complex there will always be a *releasing factor*: in the mentioned case it was the bruxism; there will also be a *local condition*: the temporal muscle on the left side was under considerable tension; and there will be a *general condition*: in this case, it was the situation at home. The problems we have to deal with in patients with disorders related to oral or occlusal dysfunction often have a general background—more or less pronounced—in which the person as a whole plays a role. The local condition is usually just one of the etiological factors, but of course sometimes a very important one.

Another example is a patient who had headaches because she was bruxing on a bridge with only a few contact spots. When she got tired of bruxing she unconsciously placed her tongue between the teeth in order to rest. During bruxing she would also clench her fist in her lap. Observing her carefully while she was clenching showed us that she would use not only elevator muscles to move the mandible and press, she also used some head positioning muscles in the neck, as well as the tongue musculature. In addition, this patient was activating the shoulder-arm-musculature. In oral and mandibular activities patients are not using just "the" temporal or just "the" masseter muscle. They always use many muscles employing different associated muscle paterns for moving the body of the mandible during oral and/or occlusal activities. It is only if we can appreciate the involved patterns of muscular activity that we can understand the dysfunctions which are connected with different types of symptoms in these patients.

Figure 2 shows the functional circle of the stomatognathic system. Since the teeth are slightly movable in their sockets, occlusal contact loading–static or dynamic–can activate periodontal receptors, apparently free branching nerve endings in the periodontal ligament. This will cause a specific sensory input to the central nervous system. In the brain many different parts may be activated, for example the reticular and the limbic systems. The resulting motor output will trigger activity of groups of jaw muscles and associated structures. Many groups of muscles must be activated at the same time in order to cause mandibular function. At the same time, muscular activity causes function of the temporomandibular joints, since they allow the movement of the mandible, and this again may cause occlusal contacts. In other words, occlusal contact activities will not only result in afferent impulses from the periodontal ligaments or other oral structures, but also from the TM-joints and from the musculature itself.

When a person bites his teeth together in the intercuspal position, the mandible comes to a stand-still because the occlusal schemes meet in such a way that the vector-sum of horizontal vectors resulting from the vertical muscular pull on the mandible will be equal to zero. In healthy stomatognathic systems this position is the end-point of a free upward swing of the mandible. If, in this situation, the occlusal schemes meet in an evenly distributed many-point-contact-pattern, then large areas of periodontal membrane are activated, and a widely distributed pattern of afferent impulses from the periodontal receptors may be expected. Under such circumstances a relative relaxation of the muscular activity around the mandible may be, and usually is, the result. This is important, because it keeps the activity level in each of the involved muscles at a state where they can be active under acceptable or "physiologic" conditions. This is the rationale behind all occlusal equilibration.

The pattern of activation of the periodontal ligament may be different when the person bites directly against a tooth, or when he moves the mandible a little, and different afferent impulse schemes may result in the two situations. This phenomenon may play

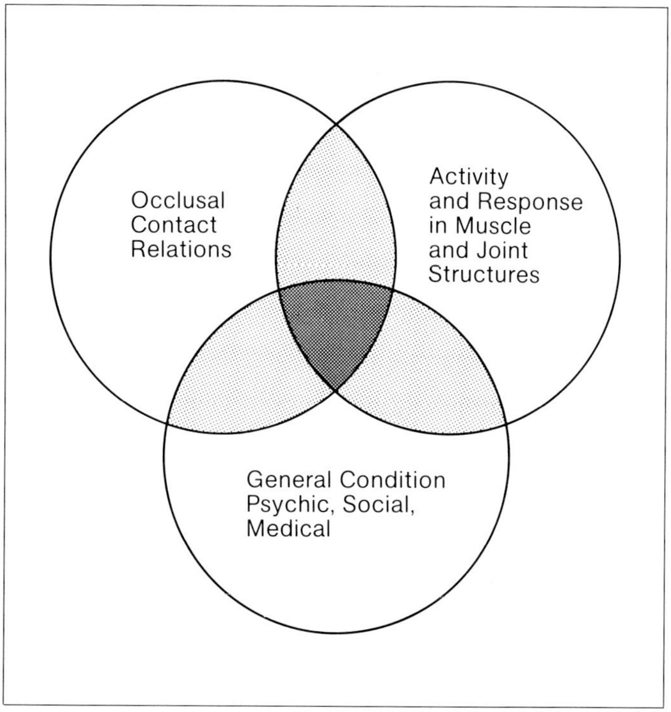


Fig. 1 Multifactorial etiology of temporomandibular function and dysfunction.

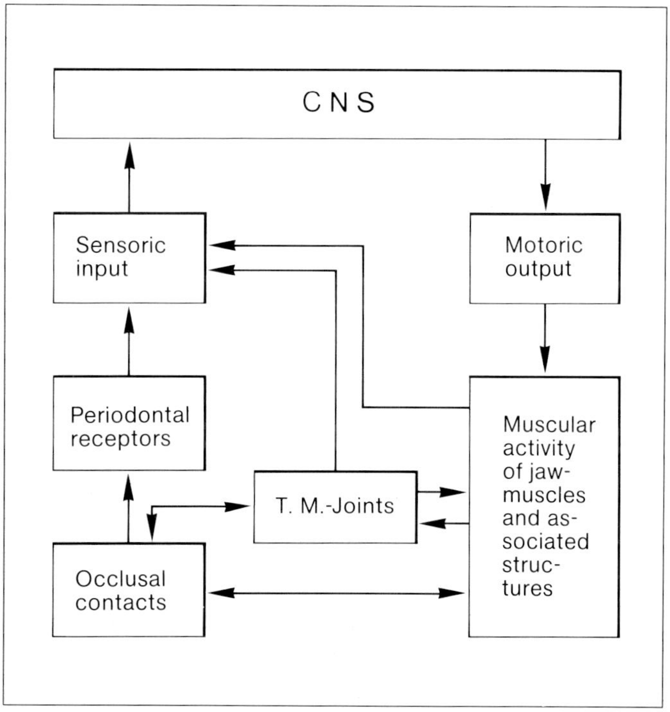


Fig. 2 Functional circle of the stomatognathic system.

a role in the forming of reflex patterns underlying oral or occlusal habits. Further, the occlusal sensibility may allow a person to discriminate very small objects, down to about 10 microns thick. In other words, even minute obstacles in the occlusal scheme may cause afferent activity from the periodontal receptors. The periodontal ligament covers all roots of the teeth like the fingers in a glove. It is thus a rather large tissue, and therefore an enormous amount of information may be released in the form of afferent impulses from the periodontal receptors. Biting at different places will alter these messages to the CNS, and in turn the CNS will alter the messages to the musculature, either causing ad hoc action or activating habitual function patterns of the mandible, the tongue, and other structures associated or coordinated with oral activities.

Under physiologic circumstances, the condition which I call *orthofunction* (Fig. 3) is characterized by a state of morphofunctional harmony mainly between occlusal morphology and the neuro-muscular function. This zone of physiologic tissue response may show a biologic variation from an ideal response to a state of adaptation. Such response is nothing more than the biochemical reactions in muscles, periodontal ligaments, TM-joints, teeth and other co-acting structures of healthy persons, when these structures are subject to biomechanical effects below a certain level of tolerance. It is a stage during which the daily activities do not cause any symptoms. Activities may go on for long periods of time with different degrees of effort and still cause response within a physiologic limit. The stage of morphofunctional harmony is thus measured by the state of physiologic tissue response. Now and then the tissues may get tired from chewing or biting, but they will soon recover after orthofunctional activity.

The term *pathofunction* does not only indicate an altered or faulty function, but also the result of such a function. In the state of pathofunction, morphofunctional disharmony is always found and it may be established in two ways.

The *morphology* of the occlusal scheme may be altered, for example through an occlusal restoration which is too high. Or the patient may have the habit of bruxing, for example on the two right canines—upper and lower. Both examples represent a morphofunctional disharmony where the morphological aspect has the primary role.

There are also morphofunctional disharmonies in which the *functional* aspect is changed. For example a stomatognathic system may work in an orthofunctional state through the years with almost no alteration of the occlusion. Then, in state of psychic stress, the general psychomotoric activity level may rise and the local occlusal contact activities increase to such a degree that a morphofunctional disharmony results. In turn, this leads to a pathologic tissue response which may occur in the TM-joints, as soft-tissue and/or hard-tissue changes (dyscrasia, prearthrotic, or arthrotic changes); the pathological tissue response may occur also in the muscles or their tendons as myofibrositis or traction-periostitis.

Between the zones of orthofunction and pathofunction there is a zone of adaptation or subliminal effects or symptoms. This situation is very common. The patients may have muscles which are sore on palpation, even if they feel no resting pain or discomfort. But the symptoms may change and become troublesome in stress situations. We have seen such a development in some dental students during the examination period. They developed pain because they were in a situation of stress. Without treatment these patients usually will recover when the examination period is over and they go on vacation.

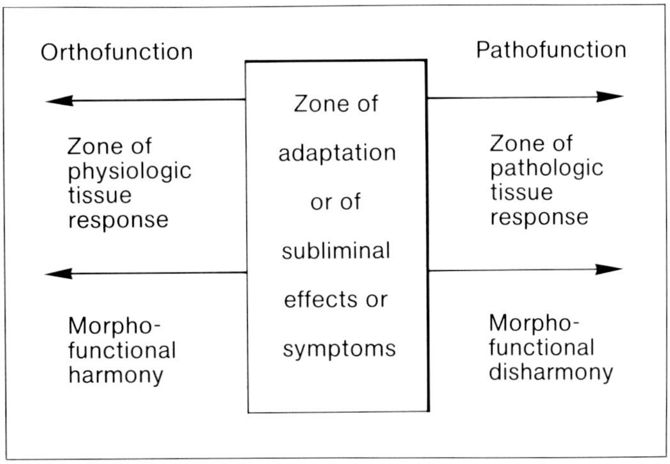


Fig. 3

It is important to have in mind that there is no distinct borderline between the healthy and the pathologic condition. In disorders related to dysfunction, the pathological situation develops gradually from the state of orthofunction to the state of pathofunction. It is our responsibility first to detect the type and location of the pathological tissue response. Secondly, we have to determine which kind of morphofunctional disharmony has caused the situation. Thirdly, we also have to judge the general psychic or social background of the patient. Our diagnosis is composed of all of these elements.

When we treat a patient, we change the pathofunctional state gradually back into a morphofunctional harmony. Thus, the way from a healthy state to disease and back again constitutes a continuum.

The pathological tissue reactions may be found in all of the tissues composing the stomatognathic system; not only in the TM-joints but also in the hard dental tissues, in periodontal tissues, in the bone, in the oral mucosa, and in muscles and tendons involved in the faulty function.

The pathological response always occurs either at the site of energy concentration, (that is, localized where forces of great intensity and long duration are active) or at sites where the tissue resistance is lowered (for example, due to an external trauma). The patho-anatomical expression of the response depends upon the structure or character of the tissue in which it occurs. However, it is characteristic for disorders related to dysfunction to occur in connective tissue or in tissues derived from the mesenchyme, such as dentine, periodontal structures, oral mucosa, bone, joint structures, interfibrillar tissue in the muscles, tendon sheaths or in the periosteum.

For example, the articular discs in Figure 4 have a perforation, or nearly so, in the lateral part. In order to visualize how these pathologic conditions might have developed, we have to realize the places where there may be a concentration of energy, i. e. a concentration of forces of considerable intensity acting over a long period of time. The lateral part of the articular disc is thinner than the medial part, that is thinner where the temporal and mandibular bony elements come closest to each other. Therefore, the lateral part of the joint is one area where energy release is likely to be concen-

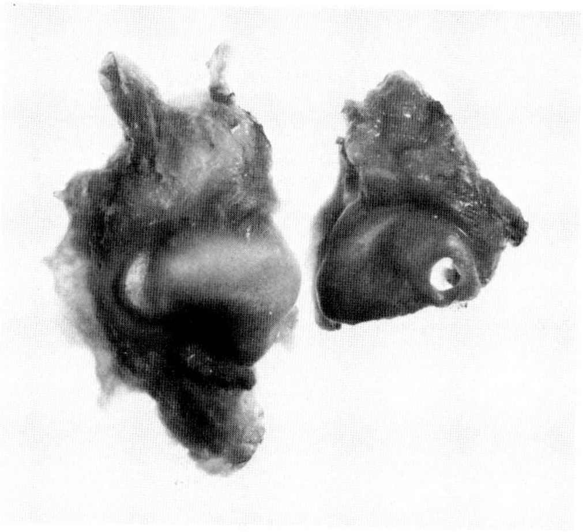

Fig. 4 Perforation of the lateral aspects of articular discs.

trated. Then there is the well-known effect of the Bennett movement-small shifts of the laterotrusive side condyle in a lateral direction when the mandible is moved to the side. This may cause soft tissues to be stained between the mandible and the temporal bone first with adaptational, and later, pathological tissue changes resulting.

In Figure 5, the traces of occlusion on a bridge are shown. When constructing the bridge the dentist apparently did not take into consideration that the patient often moves his mandible to the left and should be able to move it in a more flat path than is now possible if he follows the habitual movement pattern. So this patient started bruxing and developed a primary sliding contact on the left canine. In doing so, the right lateral pterygoid muscle contracts, causing the pathological situation which results in pain in the right TM-joint area.

This leads to a question that was brought up for discussion: Is the lateral pterygoid muscle part of the temporomandibular joint? Anatomically it is not part of the joint proper, because histologically, joint structures are characterized in one way and muscular tissues in another. Functionally, the situation is different.

In Figure 6 the temporomandibular joint is shown from the posterior aspect. The joint capsule is large and abundantly innervated. On the anterior side of the joint, the large lower and the smaller upper portion of the lateral pterygoid muscle can be seen. It is my impression that we have here two muscles which can work independently, though most often they work in close coordination with each other. The lower portion of the lateral pterygoid muscle is attached to the mandibular neck and the upper portion to the articular disc. This arrangement allows the condyle and the disc to be stabilized and to move independently, at least to some degree. They can also move or act at different speeds as in opening movements, where the condyle moves faster than the disc with the result that the disc slides backwards on to the secondary articular surface on the posterior side of the condyle in maximum opening—and vice versa in closing movements.

The arrangement as a whole also means, that when the mandible is pushed backward in a posterior border relation, tension in the posterior and lateral parts of the capsule will be created. This triggers afferent impulses which will activate the CNS and in turn, cause efferent neural impulses, some of which may

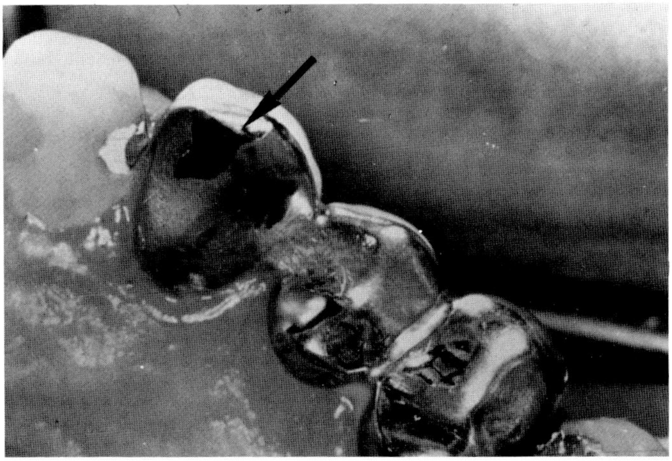

Fig. 5 Bruxofacets associated with occlusal disharmony (arrow).

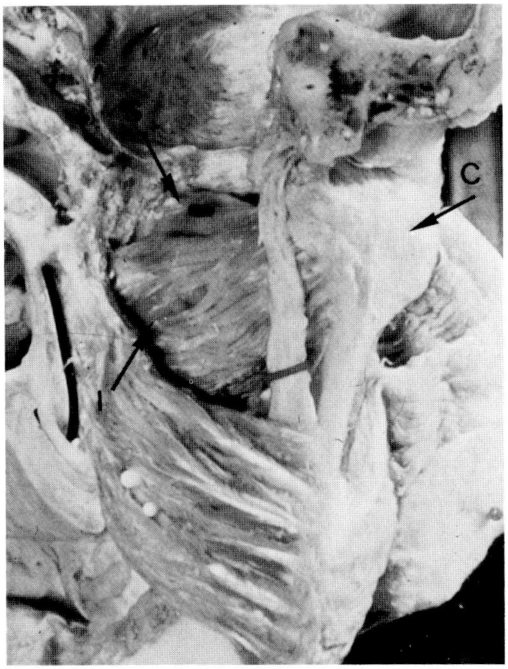


Fig. 6 Temporomandibular joint from the posterior aspect. C, joint capsule; S, upper and I, lower portion of the lateral pterygoid muscle.

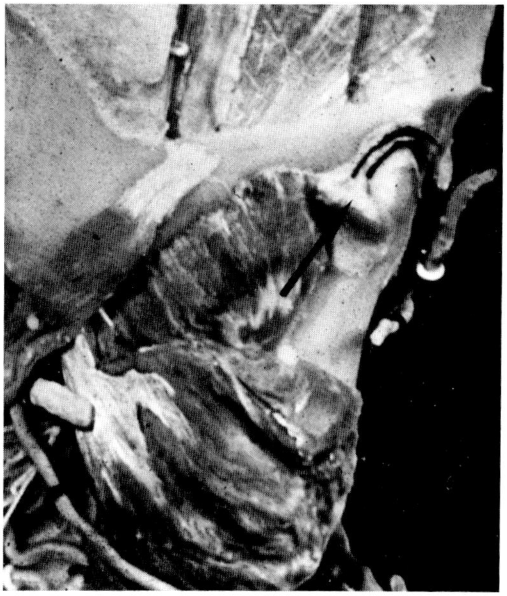

Fig. 7 Lateral ligament of the temporomandibular joint (arrow).

activate the lateral pterygoid muscles. Joints are not built to work in extreme border positions and cannot accept such an activity in the long run. They may, however, adapt to such a position through long-term changes in the tissues, but that is another story. Generally speaking, if the condyle comes into a posterior border position, this may cause a slight contraction of the lateral pterygoid muscle. Thus the lateral pterygoid muscles, the capsule, condyle, disc and other joint elements form a functional entity where the positioning of the condyle and the articular disc is due to a combination of neural and muscular activities, i. e. capsule and muscles work together via the CNS.

This is of importance in all situations where the mandible is malpositioned and we have to reposition it. The repositioning has to be done in such a way that the result is an acceptable interaction between afferent impulses from the posterior and lateral capsular structures and the slight tension of the lateral pterygoid muscle, that will keep the joint working in a morphofunctional harmony. The muscles, the joint structures and the teeth have been arranged in such a way that the form-function-equilibrium mentioned above can be maintained.

This has also to do with the lateral ligament in the joint capsule (Fig. 7). If the lateral pterygoid muscles are relaxed, and the mandible is pushed backward, the lateral ligament will become taut and thus, the backward movement stops. When it is taut, the condyle will be supported upwards by the disc, when the disc is situated in its neutral position. If the disc has become displaced forward, the condyle is supported by the loose connective tissue of the bilaminar zone. In such a case, the condyle may become displaced slightly upwards and backwards into a position where there may not exist a functional equilibrium, because the articular receptors fire in a distorted way, and consequently, may trigger muscular activity which is not in harmony with the usual patterns of the functioning occlusion. Here again, we have

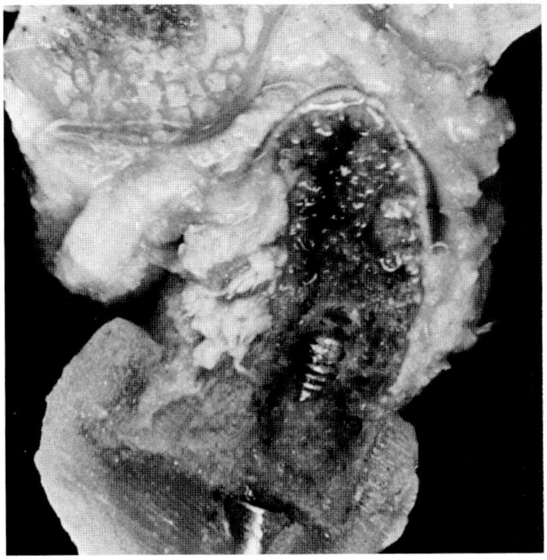

Fig. 8 Sagittal section of temporomandibular joint in neutral and/or laterotrusive position.

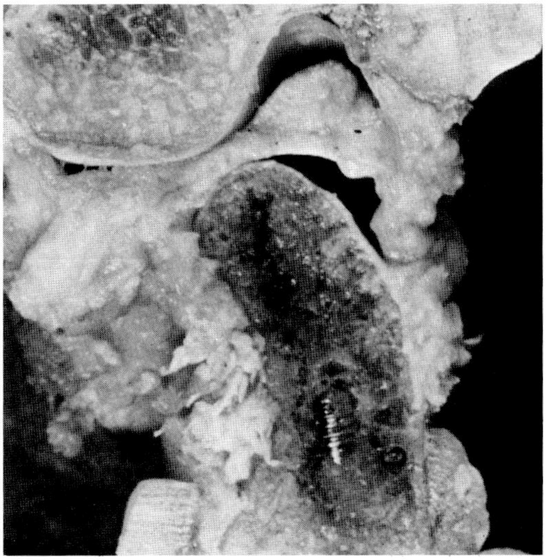

Fig. 9 Sagittal section of temporomandibular joint in slightly protrusive and/or mediotrusive position.

an example of the cooperation between form and function in nature.

Figure 8 shows a sagittal section of a TM-joint with condyle and disc. From anterior to posterior one can observe the dense part of the disc, the softer bilaminar zone, and the capsule. The condyle is supported on a surface which has a natural resilience to some degree. This is a point where a biological and a mechanical joint must deviate. Repeated efforts to position the same biological joint structure in one and the same way may result in small variations around a mean due to small deviations caused by the conditions under which the structures work in a given situation.

In a dentition with dissipated occlusal support in the intercuspal position, i. e. with full mandibular support in ICP, the teeth and the cranial pillars will, with contraction of the elevator muscles, take up the load transmitted from the mandible to the cranium, and this can generally be "accepted" by the tissues in and around the joint.

When the incisal edges make contact as in a lateral forward position of the mandible in people who brux with incisal edge-to-edge contact, the condyle of the laterotrusive (working) side is still supported in the posterior part of the joint, as seen in Figure 8, while the mediotrusive (balancing) side condyle is resting against the articular eminence (Fig. 9). This is a well supported position for a pressure transmitting joint.

The muscle which moves the condyle and disc forward is the lateral pterygoid, Figure 10. Lack of perfect coordination of the upper and lower muscle may cause displacement or subluxation of the disc, i. e. a positioning of the disc which is not in accordance with, or properly supporting, the condylar position. The important feature, therefore, is the coordination of the activity of these two muscles or parts of the muscle. But this coordination can be hampered. If a person bruxes on his right canines, he uses the upper and lower portions of the left pterygoid muscle in order to move the mandible to the right side. He also activates the elevator muscles in order to keep the canines in contact. If the two heads of this muscle are working over a long period of time and under a great load, the closing/pressing activity of the elevator muscles cause friction, and the lateral pterygoid becomes fatigued and therefore loses the fine coordination which is needed to adjust the speed of the disc to the speed of the condyle in their forward movement, as explained above. This incoordinated movement, I feel, may be one explanation of the sound caused by moving the mandible to the opposite side of the clicking joint.

After some habitual bruxing, the clicking may also happen in opening movements, since the course of movement and the difference in speed is almost the same in opening and side movements of the mandible.

Bruxing on the canines may resemble a person standing on one foot. Such a position will cause more muscular activity in the supporting leg than when he is standing on two feet. If however he stands on one foot and is able to support the position by putting his hand on a table he will again stay more stable, even with less muscular effort. That is similar to what the person in Figure 11 does. He stabilizes his mandible by means of the tongue. When the patient sits down in the dental chair and opens his mouth, the tongue drops down and backwards, and one will not be able to observe this tongue support. It can only be seen if the examiner observes the patient in an upright sitting position while talking with him. This is a clinical example of complex coordinated activity of the lateral pterygoid muscle, the elevator muscles, and the tongue musculature.

When the extrinsic tongue musculature pushes the tongue forward, there also is induced activity in the hyoid musculature. This gives us a clue to understand why patients with hyperactivity of the tongue may suffer from the so-called globulus sensation (tightening sensation in the throat, feeling of a lump in the throat). It is important to understand that we cannot treat the temporomandibular joint, or the muscles, or the occlusion as if they were separate things. It is only if we try to understand the complexity of the stomatognathic system as a whole, as well as the many activities within this system, that we can begin to realize what is going on.

The patient in Figure 12 has attrition of his front teeth. He developed this attrition without any symptoms from the joints or musculature as a gradual adaptation of the form-function-relationship. This phenomenon is seen quite often. Palpation of joints and muscles in such a case may disclose no muscle tenderness or pressure sensibility. After many years of functional harmony in the system, a bridge was constructed in the left lower molar region. The new occlusal curve was very deep with the result that the level of the last molar of the bridge became rather high. Thus the patient could only make contact on the most posterior part of that bridge in right lateral movements, and not the usual contact places in the front and/or on the laterotrusive (right) side. He could no longer use his habitual movement pattern. As soon as a patient cannot do that, he will develop a new habit resembling an attempt to "remove" the primary contact on the bridge, which hinders the habitual movements of the mandible. In turn, this means activity in the lateral pterygoid muscle on the mediotrusive (here, left) side with extended and hard work of the exposed muscle, finally resulting in pain. This leads to the conclusion that if we treat a patient who has a habitual muscular pattern which does *not* cause any pathological response, we should accept this pattern and construct any new (artificial) occlusion so as to accommodate the "well known" acceptable

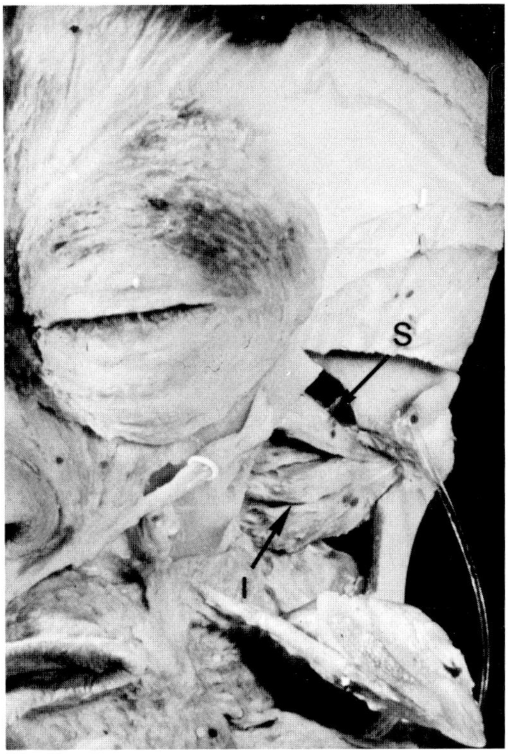


Fig. 10 Dissection of lateral pterygoid muscle. Superior (S) and inferior (I) portion of the lateral pterygoid muscle.

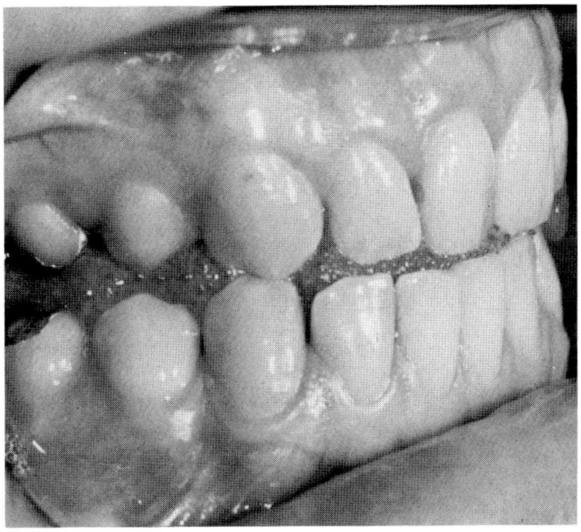

Fig. 11 Tongue stabilization in connection with bruxing on the canines.

habitual mandibular contact and movement pattern.
The occlusal activity situation mentioned above results in excess work of the left lateral pterygoid muscle and development of tension (energy concentration) in the joint area. If the place of energy concentration due to muscular force is located in this area, then it may cause structural changes—first as an adaptational, later as a pathological response—which are in accordance with the type, magnitude and duration of the forces. If, for example, the forces cause a draw on a bone, development of new bone may result. Other types of muscular activity may give rise to characteristic changes in the soft tissues. Further research may be needed in order to find out why these different types of responses develop. However, it is always mechanical factors in the form of energy concentration that will cause such development, and the tissue responses only look different in each type of tissue because the structure and mechanical and biological properties are different.
The person in Figure 5 seems to have been bruxing on his bridge "in order" to make room for lateral movements. He is what may be called an "occlusally active" patient. Had he been an "occlusally passive" patient, that is, a person whose mandible hangs in the rest position many hours a day and has little occlusal contact except during meals, then he would not be able to establish an amount of energy that would cause changes in the biological structures. It should be noted that the expressions "occlusally active" and "occlusally passive" refer to natural, acceptable mandibular activities, just as individual as any other habitual motion-pattern. If one thinks along such lines, it is possible to find a natural explanation for many hitherto not understood pathological situations that we find in patients with occlusal and oral dysfunctions.

Pathogenic lateral movements of the mandible do not necessarily occur in connection with bruxing on the teeth. Faulty function without tooth contact is also possible. A female patient claimed to have pain sensations in the TM-joints on both sides. Her pain however did not originate from the TM-joints, but from the lateral pterygoid muscles, which are in close relation to the TM-joints. In such cases the examination will disclose no pain upon digital pressure on the joints proper, from either the lateral nor the dorsal aspect, but the lateral pterygoid muscles are tender. The dysfunction of this patient involved large lateral movements of the mandible *without* tooth contact. Some patients make such movements habitually. Other common examples of faulty function without tooth contact are biting on the lips, the tongue, on hair, or on a pencil. The way in which such activities may be recognized is to observe the patients while talking with them about their problems. Activity of the tongue will cause muscular activity in the whole suprahyoid area. This, in turn, sometimes triggers off activity in the pharyngeal or laryngeal musculature, causing symptoms such as the globulus phenomenon (pharynx), or hoarseness or breathing difficulties (larynx). Often such patients have an additional symptom: a tender tongue. Usually they are not aware of that phenomenon, but squeezing the anterior part of the tongue between three fingers may disclose the condition. In patients with tongue tenderness the hyoid bone should always be palpated in order to disclose a hyperactivity of the hyoid and pharyngeal musculature.
A raised muscular activity may be found in all parts of the co-operating musculature; for example, in the head positioners or in the shoulder-arm musculature. One may also observe the suprahyoid musculature co-operating with the tongue positioner mus-

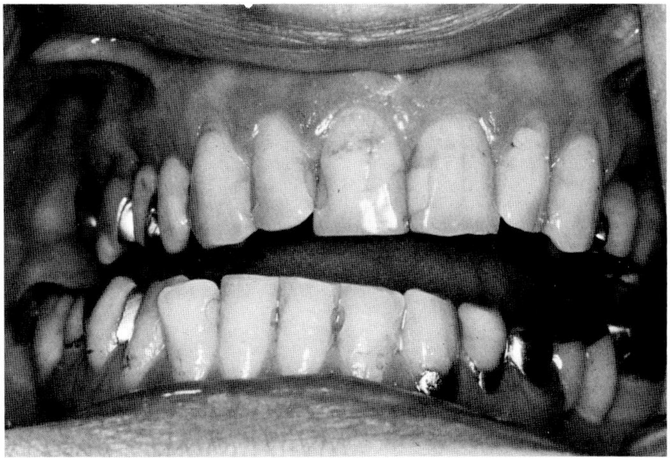

Fig. 12 Attrition in a subject judged to be in orthofunction. Further explanation in text.

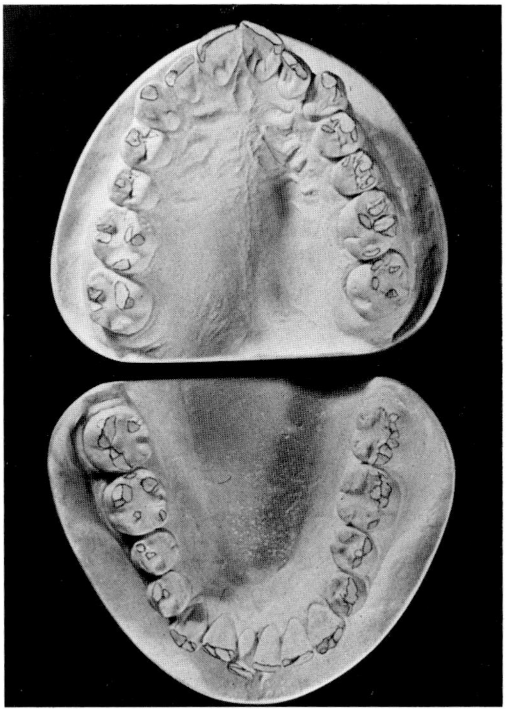

Fig. 13 Attrition facets.

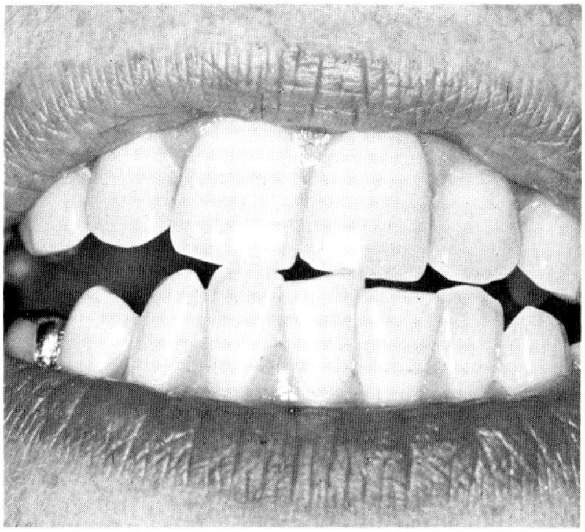

Fig. 14 Symptom-provoking tooth contact.

culature because the hyoid bone may be tilted in different ways in order to stabilize the tongue in forward, or lateral movements, or in taking any other position.

My subject today also includes some other aspects of occlusal contact activities resulting in attrition of the teeth. The many, small, flat contact areas seen in Figure 13 are a result of attrition. Usually such areas are not observed directly in the mouth because the teeth are wet. On dried-off natural teeth, or on plaster models, a pencil line may be drawn along the edge of such small facets dislosing an attrition pattern. Attrition facets may not always be single flat areas. Often they consist of several neighboring areas in different angulation to each other. This is because the facets are a result of occlusal contact activity to the right, left or forward. Such patterns may be observed on models of most young people as the result of a natural and acceptable condition. This is not in contradiction to the attempt to sometimes create an artificial occlusion without wear in accordance with certain *therapeutic* rules. Nature changes the dentition throughout life. In the beginning, the occlusal contact relations are changed through relatively fast attrition in the primary dentition and this facilitates the right positioning of the permanent teeth. Often children brux when sleeping, but I believe that most bruxing in that age happens within the state of orthofunction.

Similarly in adults, bruxing may be an occlusal activity within the sphere of orthofunction, i.e. contact movements of the teeth without so much force being exerted over so long a time that it will cause development of a pathologic tissue response. The reaction in the tissues will remain on the physiologic level. That kind of occlusal contact activity causes an adaptive attrition. Many people just touch their teeth now and then, and this activity is similar to other habitual, idle or irrelevant movements like playing with a pencil or licking the lips. Sometimes we "play" with our teeth, and this will eventually cause removal of some material from the teeth. Such rubbing of the teeth may certainly occur on the orthofunctional or adaptational level.

The contact surfaces in a given occlusal scheme are not all in use at the same time. Some are used in one movement, others in another "in order" to support the mandible in all occlusal positions and still get freedom of

movement under natural, habitual conditions.
Bruxism, in the pathophysiological sense, is not essentially different from the habitual occlusal play. It is only of longer duration and the activity of the elevator muscles is stronger. Bruxing usually consists of very short rubbing movements. Then the mandible is moved "through free air" from one contact area to the other rubbing a little here and a little there. There we find attrition facets on many different teeth and sometimes several facets on the same tooth. These facets fit together with matching facets in the opposite jaw. The mandible is moved from one place to the other, in most instances just with a touch, i. e. without development of vertical forces. Consequently the patient can brux in such positions without developing symptoms. One of these positions may be his favorite position, like the one between the right upper central and the right lower lateral incisor as shown in Figure 14. The mandible is moved a little to the left and the two facets are then fitting into each other as a key in a lock. Such a relationship is often a sign of a symptom provoking facet. In this specific mandibular position the patient may press the facets together and thus cause extra activity of the right lateral pterygoid muscle (and, of course, other muscles participating in holding that position). The symptoms will therefore be joint pain on the right side triggered off by the activity in this specific position.
If we let the patient press the teeth firmly together a short while on these facets and if they really are the symptom-provoking contact, he will soon sense his well-known symptoms. Thus, by means of this positive provocation-test, the connection between symptoms and dysfunction has been demonstrated.
In summary, it is important to realize that both diagnostic procedures and prevention of disorders due to dysfunction in the stomatognathic system depend on understanding of the working conditions of the system as a whole. We cannot talk of TM-joint disorders as a separate feature without considering the role of the occlusion, the periodontal tissues, the CNS and the musculature in the etiologic procedure, (Fig. 2). Understanding of this functional circle also gives us a clue to treatment procedures. In the dysfunctional state the functional circle has turned into a vicious ring, and this ring can be broken several ways: permanently, by changing the occlusion in such a way that the afferent impulses from the periodontal receptors are altered, or, transiently, by changing the efferent output from the CNS through psychoactive drugs or through changing the general (psychic, social, medical) background of the patient, as a whole person.

## Discussion

Discussant: Parker Mahan

*Dr. Mahan*

Well, ladies and gentlemen, what can a discusser say when he and the audience have listened to what many years of keen observations of a brilliant mind have brought to bear on the problems that you and I are concerned with here in this symposium. Dr. *Krogh-Poulsen* I don't know what to say other than, thank you so much for sharing with us the benefit of your many years experience. Dr. *Krogh-Poulsen* made his introduction by mentioning the fact that he was going to consider the variability and the response of patients to occlusal dysfunction and occlusal mutilation. Then he proceeded with the slides to do just that. He pointed out something else that I think significant in that health is more than the absence of disease; the physical, mental and social well-being of our patients should also be considered. A great start for the presentation that followed! I am proud that our profession demonstrates empathy and concern for the total patient.

Dr. *Krogh-Poulsen* spent a good deal of his time considering noxious occlusal habits and how they, through occlusal function and dysfunction, affect the temporomandibular joints, the entire stomatognathic system and ultimately the entire patient. He pointed out the adolescent patient with problems in the social realm of her life, and pointed out that going directly to the treatment of that patient's occlusion is only treating symptoms. That's a point that all of us here need to recall, that our well-meaning treatment may not be really getting at the heart of the matter. Dr. *Krogh-Poulsen*'s description of pathofunction being more than dysfunction bears mentioning again. Pathofunction, by his definition, not only includes the abnormal function, but the pathology or the tissue changes occurring as a result of that abnormality. By definition, then, pathofunction is a much more inclusive term than the more limited term, "dysfunction", as you and I might use.

Dr. *Krogh-Poulsen* pointed out that our skill as diagnosticians is based upon our ability to identify pathologic tissue responses, and he demonstrated his ability to do just that. You will recall such things as redness on the lateral sides of the lip leading him to appreciate the fact that a patient had a noxious lip-biting habit. He illustrated the principle of the dentist needing to be a keen observer of his patient if he is going to be a worthy diagnostician. He beautifully diagrammed the moments of action of the various mandibular muscles that would position a condyle. He demonstrated how we can get an abnormal position of a condyle in a radiograph and how the various muscles can be the deviating factor positioning that condyle in those abnormal positions. He spoke of the resilience of the structures in the jaw joints, and he pointed out, with specimens, the thickness of the meniscus and the fact that the TMJ is not steel. To me, he is alluding to the fact that you and I, as dentists, ought to think and function like physiologists. I think he is warning us, or stating here, that he feels that we ought to be more physiologic in our jaw registration procedures.

In my opinion he pointed out that you and I may overlook the role of the tongue and the suprahyoid muscles in the noxious habit. And then there is the tender tongue. We palpate the musculature in our patients, but how often do we palpate the tongue to determine tenderness? So a real clue here to the overall pattern of the noxious habit, is that we ought to think about the tongue and not just the elevators and the depressors of the mandible.

He mentioned the fact that we should think in terms of different responses of patients in terms of occlusion-active, as he called them, and occlusion-passive patients. That's true, isn't it? There are some people who diddle with their teeth constantly, some with a great deal of pressure, and some do this just minimally. In our diagnosing and examining of patients we need to keep that in mind. Some people have a problem because they are occlusion-active, others are so phlegmatic that they would rarely demonstrate symptoms.

Dr. *Krogh-Poulsen* pointed out that dental attrition is ubiquitous. You know people and I know people that feel that any abrasive facet on a molar is bad, and means that that patient has a problem. But Dr. *Krogh-Poulsen* has pointed out that this may be within the functional or adaptive range, or it may be in the pathologic range, and the problem we have, is to decide between the two.

Dr. *Krogh-Poulsen* demonstrated that people brux in a number of different positions. If we are going to do an occlusal adjustment, we should keep this in mind in determining how we are going to shorten or modify the length of the anterior teeth. In patients where we find these eccentric or crossover bruxing facets, we find we can get the patient to go into that position once we have directed the mandible there. Then we say "just put a little pressure there," and the patient says "ooh!" They will put their hand up and we will say, "now is that the pain we are talking about?" The patient says, "Well, yes, but I don't ever do that." I think that's diagnostic. The patient doesn't know he does it, and that's why it's a problem. One point I might make is that we have examined several TMJ's where we found lateral perforations in the meniscus, but the perforations are observed to be below the lateral lip of the mandibular fossa. These perforations at the lateral pole look to us like developmental herniations, so that the meniscus is bunched over toward the medial side. In all of these there is a three or four millimeter thick meniscus over on the medial pole of the condyle, rather than a one millimeter thick meniscus over there. It has herniated over toward the medial side. That lateral perforation was not abrasion between the lateral pole and the lateral lip of the mandibular fossa. It was apparently a developmental thing.

*Dr. Solberg*

I would like to just pursue one point Dr. *Mahan* made. I would like to direct a question to Dr. *Krogh-Poulsen* in regard to attrition. Does the natural process of attrition improve the masticatory function of the mouth or does it cause less functional efficiency?

*Dr. Krogh-Poulsen*

I don't think that it necessarily would be better or worse. If we have an attrition which is a natural attrition, as they had in the Stone Age, the occlusal surface that they developed there was excellent to chew the food that they had to chew at that time. That is beyond every doubt. In our days, with relatively little wear and tear, it is very difficult to make a generalization. I don't think it affects it very much. That is my belief.

Dr. *Solberg*

I would like to Dr. *Moffett* to make a comment please.

Dr. *Moffett*

Thank you. I just wanted to say that I think we have heard perhaps the most fundamental characterization and analysis of the biology of the stomatognathic system and of the reason why clinical management is effective, that one could ever come up with. I think we should go away from here thinking for the rest of our careers about the point that Dr. *Krogh-Poulsen* has made in regard to energy consumption, energy transformations and energy conservation. I think we can translate that so nicely to what we are doing clinically in the laboratory if we recognize that you can't have jaw function of this complexity without the consumption of energy. And I think that whenever energy is consumed, we are probably talking about a transformation that occurs between mass or form or substance and energy. The model for us is that nature is the greatest conserver of energy that we will ever see. I think that the problems that we are dealing with here are situations in which nature is giving us signals in the form of pain and other kinds of things, that this system may at times be consuming an undue amount of energy. When that happens, I think you are getting an

expensive transformation between form, structure, morphology and energy.
Clinicians empirically have discovered things that the nonclinical researchers haven't been sharp enough to see. I think Dr. *Krogh-Poulsen* has told us why we are being effective. I think we are altering, we are redistributing, we are changing energy consumption in a way which is beneficial to the patient, so that the symptoms subside. When we alter occlusion, as we have learned to do very successfully empirically, we are reducing the consumption of energy that takes place in these systems. When the nonresearcher looks at form in the laboratory and sees certain histological modifications occurring within the temporomandibular joint, he can tell where energy is being concentrated in the form of loading, compression or tension in a joint, even before there is any direct documentation of those energy exchanges. I think that Dr. *Krogh-Poulsen* has given us a preview of what the future thinking in dentistry will be.
I have to mention one other thing that makes this even more dramatic. I asked Dr. *Krogh-Poulsen* if he had been talking recently with *Melvin Moss*. He said no, and I thought that was very remarkable, because last September when I was visiting Dr. *Moss*, he told me that he will spend the rest of his career trying to take the relationships that he has identified in the functional matrix theory, and transpose them over into what he calls cellular thermodynamics. He is going to try to take the laws of thermodynamics and use them to explain the relationships that he talks about in the functional matrix. And when I hear two of my colleagues, one whom I think is the greatest contemporary nonclinical student of musculoskeletal relationships, and this morning, the world's greatest clinician researcher of this system, of its form and function, both independently arriving at exactly the same point, then I think that has tremendous significance. And I hope we can urge Dr. *Krogh-Poulsen* to put these concepts in monograph form, in the way that Dr. *Moss* is trying to do in his field. This example of two great individuals coming together and both ending up with the same concepts, may help to bridge the gap between activities in skeletal biology and what is being done in clinical dentistry today.

# VI. Surgery of the Temporomandibular Joint

by Daniel M. Laskin

## Introduction

Five to ten percent of the patients with problems involving the temporomandibular joint (TMJ) and related structures will require surgical management. Even though most of these cases are going to be treated by oral and maxillofacial surgical specialists, it is important for all dentists to have some concept of the underlying organic pathology so that they can recognize the condition, be aware of what can be done to correct the problems, and make proper referrals. My presentation will therefore discuss some of the more commonly encountered pathologic conditions affecting the temporomandibular joint, and the surgical treatments for these various conditions.

The TMJ is subject to developmental anomalies, traumatic injuries, neoplastic disease, and various forms of arthritis. These conditions are the same as those which involve other joints of the body, but they often manifest themselves differently, clinically, because the TMJ is anatomically and functionally different from most other joints. From a functional standpoint, although we talk about the temporomandibular joint, it must be remembered that the mandible is the one bone in the body which is hinged on both ends and that one joint cannot be moved independently from the other. Thus, if something alters function on one side it will simultaneously alter function on the opposite side. For this reason, pathology in one TMJ can ultimately give rise to changes in the other.

From an anatomical point of view the maxilla and the mandible are the only bones in the body that contain teeth. I will not belabor consideration of the relationship between the teeth, the musculature and the joint but only refer you to Dr. *Krogh-Poulsen*'s eloquent discussion at this symposium. The TMJ also plays an important role in growth of the mandible which we will discuss in a moment. Keeping these unique aspects of the temporomandibular joint in mind, let us proceed to the first part of my presentation.

## The role of the temporomandibular joint in mandibular growth

Because the temporomandibular joint is an area which is very important to mandibular growth, any pathologic condition that affects this joint can significantly alter this process. The growth site of the mandible is different from that of most other bones in the body because it is not protected like an epiphyseal plate; the region of growth in the TMJ is actually a part of the articulating surface. From a clinical standpoint this means that any organic pathology which involves the articulating surface in the growing individual can have a very rapid and extreme effect upon mandibular growth. This effect may be manifested in severe changes not only in growth of the mandible, but in growth of the maxilla, and even in the entire cranial complex.

*Sarnat* and others before him have demonstrated that if you do a condylectomy on a growing animal, there will be a very characteristic change in the morphology of the mandible. Based on this work, the mandibular condyle was considered as a primary growth center for the mandible. However, in 1971, *Sarnat* did a similar condylectomy study in a group of animals that were already grown. These new studies demonstrated that qualitatively but not quantitatively the changes found in the animals that had stopped growing were the same as those in the animals that were still growing. It suddenly became obvious that the mandibular condyle was not a primary growth center and that perhaps *Moss* was correct when he talked about the functional matrix being the driving force behind mandibular growth. *Moss* suggested that the mandibular condyle really serves as a secondary growth site which adapts to the changes that accompany growth of the soft tissue structures.

My own subsequent experiments on the role of condylar growth tend to support this concept. These experiments involved three series of monkeys, each including both a young and an old group. In the first series we repeated *Sarnat*'s experiment by doing a condylectomy. The second series of animals had an ostectomy in the ramus of the mandible to lower the condyle. This procedure resulted in the same amount of ramal shortening as with condylectomy, but maintained the potential for growth of the condyle in the young animals. In the third series, a condylectomy was done in young and old animals but the condyle was replaced with an artificial prosthesis. These experiments demonstrated that condylectomy produces similar results in both the young and old animals, which is what *Sarnat* told us in 1971. In the animals where the condyle was still present, though lowered by ostectomy, we found that the changes in the young animals were minimized. In the adult animals, the same changes were produced as in the condylectomy group. These results indicated that the condyle does have a growth potential but it didn't answer the question as to whether it is primary or secondary. The third experimental series demonstrated that the implant does minimize the changes in the young animal but does not eliminate them; in the old animals the implants prevented the changes. The logical conclusion from these experiments is that the mandibular condyle is an important area of growth, but that it is a secondary growth site which tends to compensate for the downward and forward movement of the mandible that is brought about by what *Moss* refers to as growth of the functional matrix. The implications of this concept in clinical diagnosis and treatment will become apparent as we proceed with the next part of this discussion.

## Pathologic conditions involving the TMJ

### Agenesis

Agenesis can be found in hemifacial microsomia (First arch syndrome), and in Goldenhar's syndrome. These syndromes all exhibit a partial to total absence of the temporomandibular joint. Agenesis can also involve part of the mandibular ramus as well as portions of the inner and outer ear and other structures on the side of the face (Fig. 1).

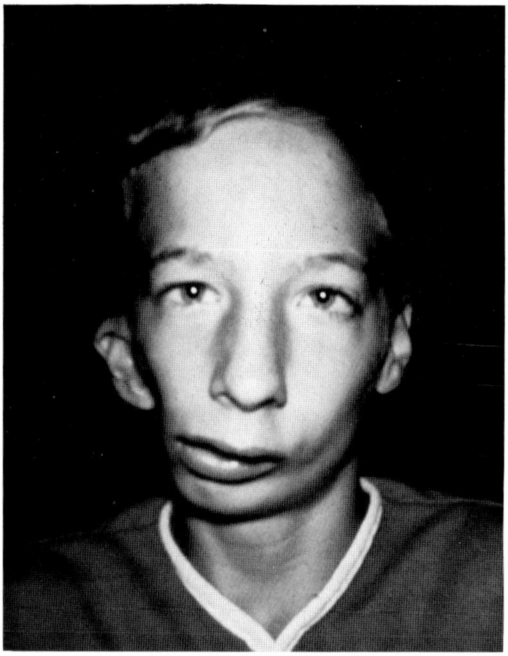

Fig. 1 Nine-year-old patient with hemifacial microsomia.

a) Frontal view showing severe facial deformity with mandible deviated to the affected side.

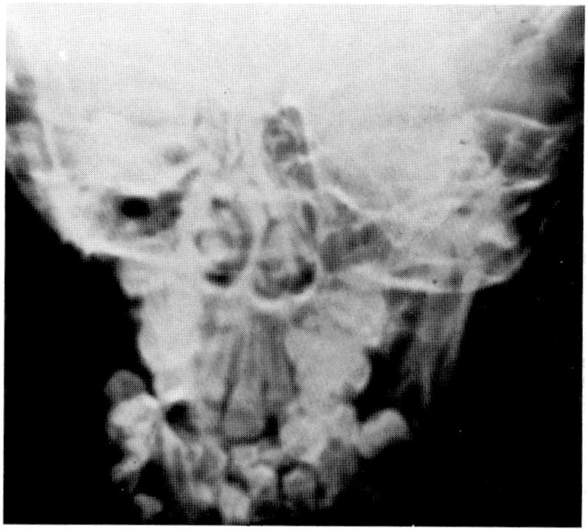

b) Radiograph shows absence of body and ramus of the mandible distal to the second molar. (From Diseases of the Temporomandibular Joint by Daniel M. Laskin, Chapter 12, in Oral Surgery, edited by James R. Hayward, Charles C. Thomas, Publisher, Springfield, Ill., 1976).

Patients with unilateral agenesis, or any other form of unilateral mandibular growth arrest, will exhibit a very characteristic appearance, with a long face on one side, and a short face on the other. There is usually a severe malocclusion (retrognathia) which indicates that even though the condyle is not a primary growth site it does have a significant effect upon occlusal development. When the mouth is opened there is a tendency for a deviation of the mandible to the affected side.

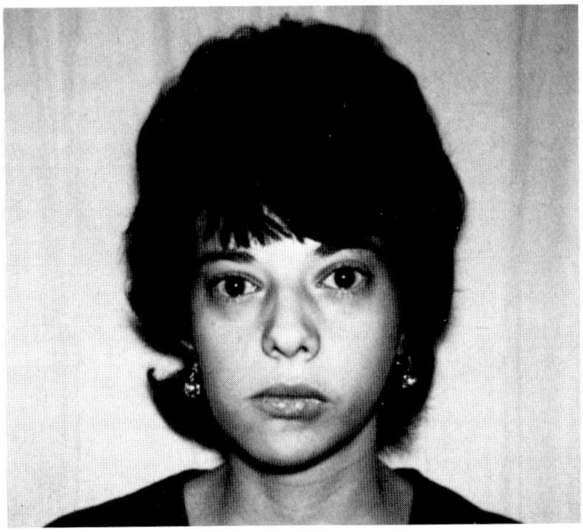

Fig. 2 Twenty-year-old patient with condylar hypoplasia resulting from injury at age six. The normal side of the mandible (left) is longer and flatter than the affected side.

Treatment: The first consideration in surgical treatment of agenesis is to provide some sort of mechanical strut for the mandible so that any facial growth taking place will not be unidirectional but will be as symmetrical as we can possibly make it. The second thing that we would like to do is replace the missing condyle with some tissue which has a potential for continued growth. Since, ideally, the mechanical strut should be able to increase in size as the patient grows, it is necessary to use a biologic material. I prefer to use a rib graft (costochondral junction) rather than some of the other biologic tissues that have been tried. The third recommendation I would like to make for the surgical treatment of agenesis is that the grafting procedure be done early to provide direction to whatever growth is occurring. Unless there is sufficient functional matrix, however, a second or third operation may be necessary to maintain a continued symmetrical appearance and proper mandibular function.

**Unilateral condylar hypoplasia**

A less serious involvement of the temporomandibular joint than agenesis is unilateral condylar growth arrest, or condylar hypoplasia. This condition can be congenital in origin, although most often it is post-traumatic. It produces the same qualitative changes in form as occur in those patients with agenesis but not the same quantitative changes. Patients with hypoplasia will exhibit condylar deformity, a short-wide ramus, shortening of the body of the mandible, antegonial notching, and fullness of the face on the affected side (Fig. 2). On the unaffected side there will be a relative elongation of the mandibular body and flatness of the face. There is generally a Class II malocclusion due to the mandibular underdevelopment. These findings become important in establishing a differential diagnosis between unilateral condylar hypoplasia and unilateral condylar hyperplasia. With facial asymmetry it can be very difficult to decide whether you have a patient that is exhibiting overgrowth on one side or an underdevelopment on the other side.

Treatment: Treatment of unilateral condylar hypoplasia is going to depend upon the individual case, what the occlusion is like, and the degree of facial deformity. Sometimes the mandible is lengthened on the short side;

sometimes the normal side will be shortened. Age is an important consideration in the treatment of unilateral condylar hypoplasia—whether it is congenital or post-traumatic in origin. Treatment should take place before the active growth period ends to be most effective. The clinical features of untreated unilateral hypoplasia in a child are going to manifest themselves early. In fact, at six or seven years of age you will begin to notice the patient's face becoming asymmetrical. The problem will get worse as time goes on, and it gets more difficult to achieve a good cosmetic result. With a bilateral hypoplasia, even though you may get a deformity, it is symmetrical. It is always much easier to correct a symmetrical deformity than an asymmetrical one, so the timing of treatment is less critical in the former situation.

### Unilateral condylar hyperplasia

Unilateral condylar hyperplasia is the opposite condition to condylar hypoplasia. It is characterized by an enlargement of the condyle which is symmetrical, and histologically there is no real pathologic abnormality in the progression of cartilage into bone. If there is an asymmetrical condyle, aberrant patterns of endochondral bone formation, and excessive cartilage formation, one is generally dealing with a condylar tumor (chondroma, osteochondroma) rather than a hyperplasia. Sometimes the condyle isn't enlarged but the neck merely tends to become elongated. The body and the ramus on the affected side often are also elongated, but no antegonial notching is present. If the condition occurs early in the individual's development, you will find a bowed appearance of the lower border. The lower border becomes rounded because, as the mandible is displaced away from the maxilla, there is a tendency for the teeth to erupt in an attempt to maintain occlusion thereby causing an increase in the height of the alveolar process. On the unaffected side, there is a normal size body and ramus. Skeletally and dentally, patients will have either a Class I, or, more frequently, a tendency toward a Class III relationship with a prominent chin (Fig. 3).

Treatment: With condylar hyperplasia, the factors of occlusion, skeletal tendencies and facial deformity are important considerations in treatment. In addition, it is important to know if the condyle is still growing, and this can be determined with serial cephalometric radiographs and bone scans. If you have a patient with a severe unilateral condylar hyperplasia which is still growing, treatment should consist of condylectomy. If the condyle is no longer growing, corrective surgery can be done on other parts of the mandible. In either instance, sufficient bone is removed to permit symmetrical repositioning of the mandible.

### Condylar tumors

Although malignant tumors occur, most tumors involving the TMJ are benign and our discussion will be limited to this group. The most frequent tumor is the osteochondroma. Patients with benign condylar tumors often look quite similar to patients with condylar hyperplasia yet, as previously stated, there are characteristic differences. One major difference is in condylar morphology, where a tumor will generally produce an asymmetrical condyle (Fig. 4). Very rapidly growing tumors of the condyle will also cause a unilateral posterior open bite because the teeth do not have sufficient opportunity to erupt and come into contact. In more slowly growing tumors, you will find that the teeth will maintain occlusion of some sort and there will be a greater tendency to bowing of the lower border of the mandible.

Treatment: Treatment of benign condylar

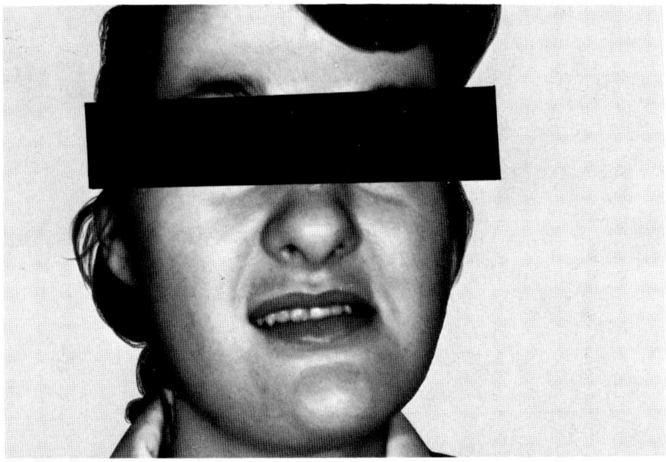

Fig. 3a

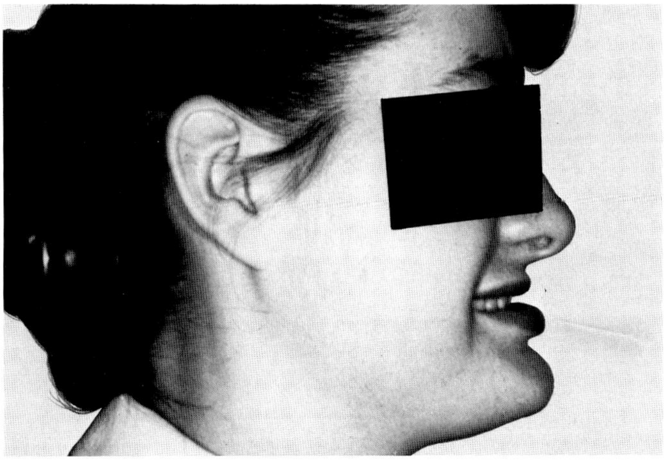

Fig. 3b

Fig. 3c

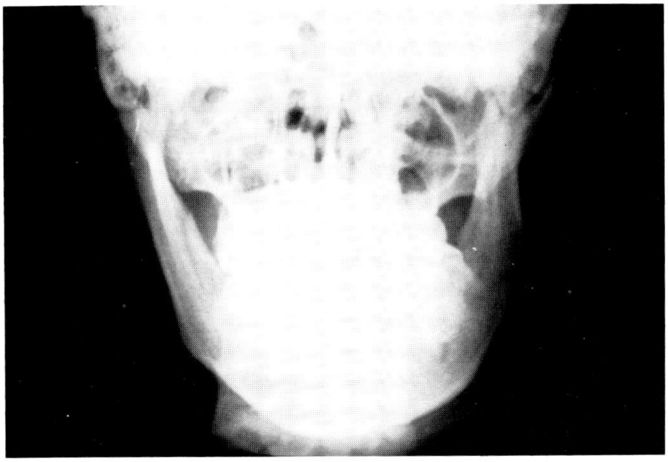

Fig. 3 Patient with unilateral condylar hyperplasia showing increased length of right side of mandible, crossbite malocclusion and prognathic appearance. The face is flatter on the abnormal side. (From B. G. Sarnat and D. M. Laskin, Diagnosis and Surgical Management of Diseases of the Temporomandibular Joint, Charles C. Thomas, Publisher, 1962).

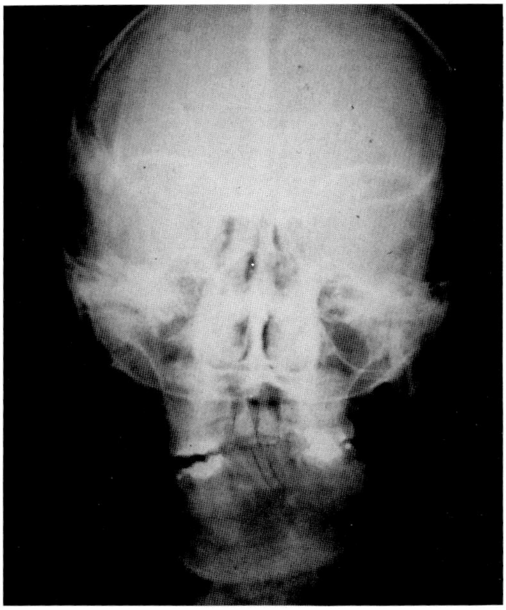

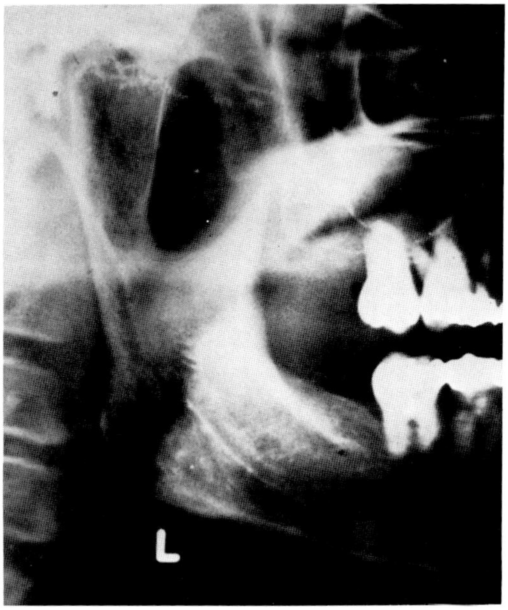


Fig. 4 Radiographs of patient with osteochondroma of mandibular condyle.

a) Frontal views showing similarity to radiograph of patient with unilateral condylar hyperplasia in Figure 3.

b) View of condyle showing abnormal morphology. Separation of the teeth on the right side indicates that lesion is rapidly growing.

tumors usually involves removal of the lesion and shortening of the mandible on the affected side if it is elongated. Patients with condylar tumors often have the same prognathic tendency as patients with hyperplasia, and surgical treatment generally yields a good cosmetic result.

## Dislocation

A dislocation, by definition, is a derangement between the articulating components of a joint that is not self-reducing. I would like to emphasize that definition and distinguish it from a subluxation, which I would define as a self-reducing derangement between the articulating components of a joint that is associated with symptoms of pain, clicking or momentary locking. Radiographically, the position of the condyle relative to the articular eminence is not very diagnostic of subluxation since there have been several studies that have shown that a normal individual can move the condyle as far as 5 mm in front of the articular eminence. Therefore, only patients who additionally exhibit pain, clicking, and momentary locking should be classified as having subluxation. This distinction has not been made clear in the literature, and therefore much confusion exists about the surgical management of these conditions. I seriously question whether surgical treatment is frequently indicated for the clinical situation where a patient has only temporary locking, clicking and momentary deviation on opening. I want to emphasize that I am going to be discussing *dislocation* of the mandible and not subluxation.

What are the factors which lead to a patient developing chronic recurrent dislocation? First, an individual who normally has a wide opening range is a good candidate for occurrence of this situation. Another possible predisposing factor is laxity or looseness of the capsule and ligaments. In addition to these predisposing factors, something must initiate the dislocation. Dislocation is usually caused by sudden wide opening, or it can be initiated by prolonged wide opening such as might occur during dental treatment.

Acute dislocations of the mandible which do not recur are really not surgical problems. However, chronic recurrent dislocation and chronic persistent dislocation of the mandible are surgically treatable conditions. Chronic persistant dislocation can occur when a patient dislocates and is not reduced for a number of weeks, or sometimes even months. I am not going to discuss this problem in detail except to say it occurs rarely and surgery is probably indicated to correct it.

Assuming a patient has both the predisposing factors and the initiating incident, what is the mechanism of recurrent dislocation of the mandible? It is important to understand this because if you don't understand etiology there is no way to rationally treat the resultant condition. There are two major concepts about what causes dislocation. One states that the condyle translates beyond the articular eminence and is mechanically prevented from returning to the fossa. The other states that the dislocation is maintained by muscular spasm. As with every controversial issue, there are the "fence sitters" who say it is a combination of these two factors. Personally, I belong to the second school of thought which says that dislocation is due to masticatory muscle spasm.

It is difficult to conceive how the concept of mechanical blockage arose. It is probably related to the fact that we generally think about the TMJ in a lateral projection. From a lateral view the structure we see hanging down is not the articular eminence but rather the articular tubercle, which is the structure to which the temporomandibular ligament is attached. If you take a human skull, turn it over, and look at it from the bottom you will find that the eminence has a posterior slope but little or no anterior slope. The area beyond the crest of the eminence is relatively flat and it isn't really mechanically possible for this area to have much of a blocking effect. Another factor that possibly contributes to the confusion is that we are taught to treat dislocation by pushing down on the mandible, to get it under the eminence, and then moving it backward. Now I grant you that downward pressure on the mandible works, but you push it down not to get the condyle under the eminence but to stretch the shortened muscles. In a hyperextended state it is the direction of pull of the spastic jaw-closing muscles that tends to maintain the dislocation.

Treatment: Treatment of chronic recurrent dislocation has involved both nonsurgical and surgical methods. One method is mandibular immobilization, which is fine for a patient who has dislocated once, or maybe twice, and there is a tearing of the tissues. In this situation, if you immobilize the mandible there is capacity for repair. In patients that have dislocated 10 or 20 times, however, everything is so loose that they do not tear very much tissue when they dislocate and you could immobilize them for long periods of time and nothing is going to happen. Mandibular immobilization is, therefore, not a good treatment for people with chronic recurrent dislocation. The other nonsurgical treatment is the injection of a sclerosing agent into the capsule or into the TMJ ligament which produces an inflammatory response and gives rise to fibrosis and tightening of these structures. Injection of sclerosing agents is considered a relatively noninvasive technique. However, caution must be used with this procedure because you run the risk of producing degenerative changes in the synovium, and those structures which derive nutrition from the synovium, if you inject directly into the joint space rather than into the ligament and capsule.

In addition to the nonsurgical techniques, there are also at least 5 major surgical methods which have been recommended:

1. Tightening of the capsule by plication or excision of a portion of the capsule
2. Anchoring of the mandible to adjacent structures
3. Mechanical blockage of condylar movement
4. Removal of interferences to condylar movement
5. Reduction of muscle pull

The first thing that should come into your mind when you see a list of five different categories of operations, with two or three operations in each category, is that no one procedure provides all the answers. If one method was very successful there would only be one recommended operation, not five different categories. If you look at the literature, you will find that tightening the capsule, mechanical blockage and removal of interferences have all been reported as giving good results. However, those cases where the mandible was anchored to adjacent structures did not seem to have the same good results. Since several diverse procedures are reported to be effective, the logical conclusion is that there is something common to these operations. Probably the common factor is that they are all intraarticular procedures that produce scarring of the capsule and ligament. Since scarring of the tissues is curative for most patients, this can be accomplished just as effectively, and more safely, by injection of a sclerosing agent than by surgical intervention. For those patients in whom the etiologic factors are still active, however, the joint will soon become hypermobile again. For such cases I have recommended an operation called lateral pterygoid myotomy. I use this operation very sparingly, and generally most of the patients on whom I have done this operation have been epileptics where you cannot control the seizures pharmacologically. These patients will continue to have seizures and they will loosen the joint again and again. Mentally retarded patients, patients who have other mental problems, or patients with orofacial dyskinesia who exhibit excessive mandibular gyrations are also possible candidates for the myotomy procedure.

The basis for this operation is the idea that if you detach the lateral pterygoid muscle you change the opening movement from hinge and glide to only a hinge movement, and the patient will not dislocate any longer. This operation basically involves detachment of the lateral pterygoid muscle. After detaching the muscle, a piece of Silastic is placed in front of the neck of the condylar process to prevent the muscle from reattaching. This treatment seems to work very well in those patients where other forms of therapy have failed.

## Ankylosis

Ankylosis can be defined as a limitation of motion due to pathologic involvement of the joint. It is not really a disease in the true sense; it is rather a symptom of many diseases. It can result from trauma, rheumatoid arthritis, or from congenital problems. Ankylosis is different from trismus or from the limitation of movement associated with the MPD syndrome, which are both muscular phenomena. Ankylosis can be classified as true or false, and bony or fibrous. False ankylosis produces limitation by involving other parts of the mandible than the temporomandibular joint.

Facial deformity and ankylosis do not necessarily go together. When they do occur simultaneously it is because the process which is producing the ankylosis is also destroying the growth tissue on the head of the condylar process. Any pathologic process in the joint can have this same effect. If you have a false ankylosis it will produce just as much limitation as a true ankylosis but it will have no effect upon facial growth since the condyle is not involved. Radiographically, bony ankylosis will show a loss of the normal architecture making it impossible to distinguish between condyle and glenoid fossa and zygomatic arch. Ability to partially open the mouth does not always indicate a fibrous ankylosis. Even with bony ankylosis the patient can sometimes open the mouth as much as a centimeter due to elasticity of the bone.

Treatment: There are five basic principles involved in the treatment of ankylosis of the temporomandibular joint. First, all patients with ankylosis should be operated on as early as possible. As pointed out previously, the important thing is to obtain jaw movement to give the functional matrix an opportunity to express itself in terms of mandibular growth. By being treated early, these patients will become less asymmetrical than if you leave them alone and wait, and wait, and wait, before you operate on them. Second, every effort should be made to maintain the height of the ramus or otherwise the surgery will cause additional facial deformity. Third, union of the parts after surgery must be prevented. Fourth, in a growing individual we should replace the lost growth center with a biologically compatible growing tissue (Fig. 5). Finally, it is essential to maintain an active program of jaw-stretching exercises, postoperatively, to prevent scarring which would result in reduced opening.

The surgical approach to ankylosis in the adult involves creation of a new joint as close to the old joint area as possible so as to maintain height of the ramus. One should never operate in the middle of the ramus if the procedure can be performed close to the glenoid fossa. Ramal height in a nongrowing individual can be maintained with any biocompatible material. Silastic is commonly used. It is generally fastened to the stump of the condylar process. If this is not possible, it is fastened to the zygomatic arch to create a cushion upon which the lower part of the mandible can function. Even though a bilateral procedure will not produce jaw asymmetry, it can lead to an anteriorly opened bite. If you want to avoid this situation in bilateral ankylosis cases you have to maintain height of the ramus.

Ankylosis in the growing individual requires a different treatment than in the adult. The longer you wait with a unilateral problem the more asymmetrical the face becomes, the more the occlusion is affected, and the greater the difficulty in achieving a reasonably successful end result. Therefore, these patients should always be operated early, and a biological tissue should be inserted. A costochondral junction will not only provide a growing patient with replacement of what is missing, but it will also provide the potential for additional growth to occur (Fig. 5). In addition, using growing cartilage as a joint replacement is advantageous since it will not fuse to the bony parts and will therefore prevent re-ankylosis.

Functional rehabilitation after surgery of the TMJ is also extremely important to achieve good results. Not only do you have scarring and fibrosis of the joint after surgery, but usually some atrophy or shortening of the muscles is present before surgery. By a program of proper exercises it should be pos-

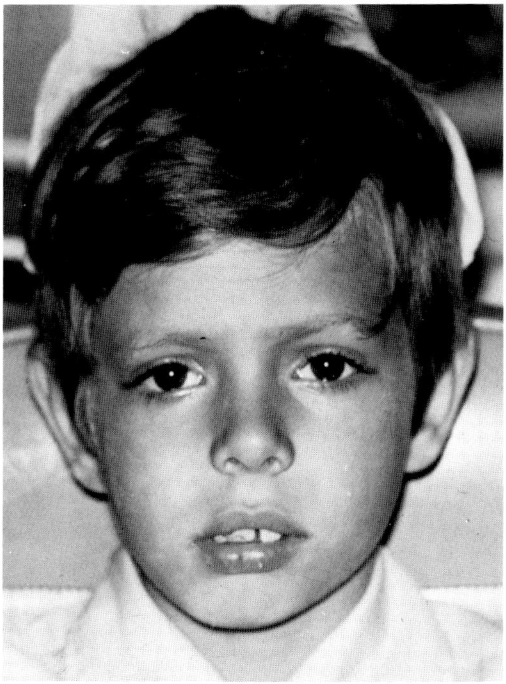

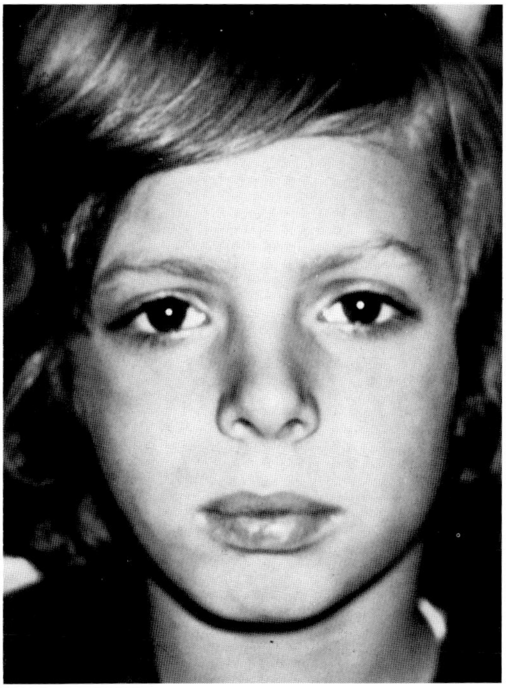

Fig. 5

a) Six-year-old child with unilateral ankylosis resulting from fracture of condyloid process. Note the facial asymmetry.

b) Child at age nine, three years after correction of ankylosis and insertion of costochondral graft to replace the condyle. Symmetrical growth of mandible has occurred resulting in correction of facial deformity.

sible to maintain, or even improve, the degree of opening achieved at the time of surgery.

## Rheumatoid arthritis

Rheumatoid arthritis (RA) is characterized by intermittant pain, swelling, and limitation of movement that is progressive. After an acute episode of RA the limitation in jaw opening will improve a little bit but it is a downhill pattern. RA commonly involves other body joints first, but the temporomandibular joint is ultimately involved in at least 50% of these cases, if not more. In some instances, rheumatoid arthritis is recognized first in the temporomandibular joint. It is usually a bilateral involvement, although it may start in one joint.

In addition to joint involvement, there are the associated phenomena of the generalized disease process such as anemia, fever, malaise and anorexia. Blood examination will usually yield positive laboratory findings in the acute phase of the condition, although sometimes it is difficult to get positive tests in a remission stage. The radiographic changes which occur in RA are relatively late in the course of the disease. That is because RA is a primary disease of the soft tissues and soft tissue changes, as Dr. *Öberg* pointed out, are not recognizable initially. As the

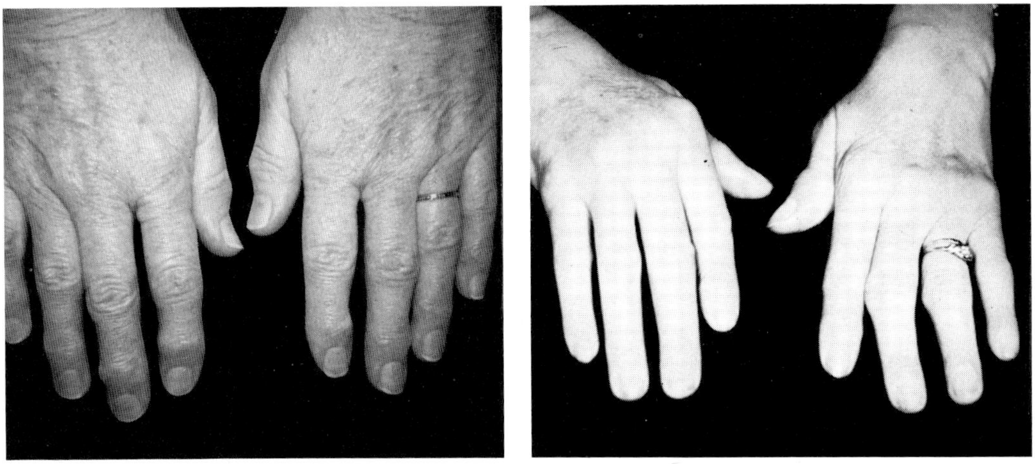

Fig. 6 Manifestations of arthritis in the hands. Top, Osteoarthritis. Note the bony enlargement of the terminal interphalangeal joints (Heberden's nodes). Bottom, Rheumatoid arthritis. The hands are more deformed, with deviation of several fingers. The major area of involvement is the proximal interphalangeal joint, causing the fingers to have a fusiform appearance.

synovial tissues become more involved, pannus formation takes place, and destructive enzymes are secreted; then you begin to get bony erosions which can be seen on the radiographs.

Whenever rheumatoid arthritis of the TMJ occurs in a young individual it is going to have an effect upon facial growth. In an older patient this is not an important consideration.

One of the earliest symptoms of RA in the adult patient, in addition to pain in the temporomandibular joint, is the inability to bring the incisors into occlusion. RA patients characteristically develop an anteriorly opened bite because of the fact that they have destruction of the condylar surfaces which results in a progressive loss of height of the mandibular rami.

In addition to the anterior open bite, there is a characteristic appearance of the hands of a rheumatoid arthritis patient which is different from that in degenerative arthritis patients. There is a tendency for the middle phalanx to become involved and for spindle shaped fingers to develop which are wide at the knuckle and taper toward the end of the finger. As the condition progresses the fingers tend to skew in various directions (Fig. 6). By contrast, degenerative or osteoarthritis tends to involve the terminal phalanx, so instead of getting enlargement at the knuckle, the finger gets knobby just adjacent to the fingernail. Also, the fingers remain relatively straight. These differences can sometimes be helpful as an aid to differential diagnosis in the older individual.

Treatment: Over time, the condition of RA gets progressively worse and, in the child, a significant facial deformity results. Unfortunately, we do not have very many answers regarding the treatment of rheumatoid arthritis, at least from a surgical standpoint. The primary management of rheumatoid arthritis is medical. Only when, and if, the condition gets severe enough to produce ankylosis does surgical management become part of treatment. If the RA process is no longer active, the patient is treated in a manner similar to any patient with ankylosis that is post-traumatic, except that in a young patient costochondral grafts should be avoided since they may resorb if the arthritis again becomes active. For the patient where you are unsure of the state of remission, the additional precaution of completely covering the articulating surface, rather than merely interposing an alloplastic material, should be taken because recurrence of the ankylosis due to the inflammatory tissue growing around the site of correction can occur if there is recrudescence of the condition.

## Degenerative joint disease

The condition which is perhaps the most common pathologic problem involving the TMJ, degenerative arthritis, will be my final topic of discussion. The most controversial aspect of this disease is whether one should adopt an approach which is nonsurgical or whether one should use surgery. As an aid in making this decision, I prefer to consider degenerative arthritis in two main categories, primary and secondary. From a histopathologic standpoint, there is perhaps no difference between the two groups, but from the clinical standpoint there is an obvious difference in symptoms and possibly etiology. Primary degenerative arthritis is relatively asymptomatic; the condyle may show flattening and lipping, and the patient will have crepitation, but he won't come to the office complaining of it. Most often, primary degenerative arthritis of the TMJ is observed as part of a general evaluation of a patient for some other condition. From an etiologic standpoint it can be considered to be part of the natural wear and tear, and aging process of the individual. As anyone gets older, usually in the late fifties, sixties or seventies, he begins to show some asymptomatic arthritic changes in the temporomandibular joint.

Secondary degenerative arthritis is generally seen in a slightly younger age group (20–40) and I believe it is a phenomenon which follows the myofascial pain-dysfunction (MPD) syndrome. The MPD syndrome represents a process which initially starts in the musculature but if prolonged it can secondarily involve the TMJ. Patients with secondary degenerative arthritis complain of pain, crepitation, and muscle tenderness, clicking or hypomobility. You will see radiographic changes which are similar but often not as severe as those in patients with primary degenerative arthritis. Probably there is less radiographic change because the more severe symptoms lead to earlier recognition of the condition.

Secondary degenerative arthritis, like RA, exhibits intermittent acute phases. The painful symptoms initially represent myofascial pain, not articular pain. Subsequently, if patients begin to get erosions, spurring and other articular changes, the painful symptoms actually represent pain coming from the TMJ as well as from the associated musculature.

Treatment: There are basically four different types of operations that have been recommended for treatment of degenerative arthritis. Here, as with dislocation, since there is more than a single method one must look critically at the recommended procedures.

First, if you examine the literature, one of the earliest operations recommended was meniscectomy. *Bowman* reported a large series of cases where he had used meniscectomy and concluded that it was not an ideal treatment for degenerative arthritis. Once you did a meniscectomy, you were creating an opportunity for degenerative changes to become even worse because of loss of the normal cushioning effect of the disc.

The second operation which was recom-

mended is the condylectomy, which by definition is the removal of the entire head of the condyloid process. It is an unfortunate situation that reports of some techniques tend to be rushed into print, but we fail to see reports when the individuals who devised the operations are no longer using them. When a resident or practitioner searches the literature, and reads about a technique which sounds good, he will then go through the same mistakes that have already been made. At one time condylectomy was used, but it is now no longer recommended because it can produce more problems then the original disease.
The third operation, condylotomy, is an outgrowth of the condylectomy procedure. This operation makes a little more sense because it involves only the partial removal of the condyle and at least you are maintaining most of the height of the ramus as well as the attachment of the lateral pterygoid muscle. If the pathology is severe enough to require surgical removal then I believe that it is perfectly legitimate to do a condylotomy. However, I personally prefer a fourth procedure called an arthroplasty. Arthroplasty is a broad term which actually means the reconstruction of a joint. However, in the context generally used for TMJ surgery it implies removal of only enough bone to eliminate any spurring, lipping or erosion.
What are the indications for arthroplasty? First, the elimination or treatment of all extra-articular pathology. Second, the patient must be psychologically stable. Third, I only operate after a patient has had no response to conservative therapy. In other words, these patients have to have a fair try on all of the things that are normally helpful to such patients. These conservative measures include bite-plates, medications and re-establishment of a well functioning dentition. Lastly, I would also like to have some radiographic evidence of degenerative joint disease. In the past this meant bony change, but now with the revived use of arthrograms perhaps we will be able to establish some definitive evidence of joint changes involving soft tissue, and our indications for surgery and the types of procedures used may eventually be modified. As a general rule, it is always important to attempt all nonsurgical methods before considering surgery for degenerative arthritis.

## Summary

Surgery has a very specific place in the management of certain conditions involving the temporomandibular joint. These include developmental anomalies, traumatic injuries, recurrent and persistent dislocations, the sequelae of some forms of arthritis, ankylosis and neoplastic disease. However, because the more common conditions, such as myofascial pain-dysfunction (MPD) syndrome and degenerative arthritis, generally produce similar signs and symptoms, but usually do not require surgery, the ability to establish a correct diagnosis is essential. When this is accomplished, surgical treatment can resolve many of the TMJ problems encountered.

## Discussion

Discussant: William McCarty

First of all, Dr. *Laskin*, let me say that I really enjoyed your talk. I only disagree on one aspect of your presentation, and that is your claim that only 10% of patients with TMJ disorders require surgery. In Montgomery I have found the percentage closer to 18%. I would like to agree with several aspects of your presentation such as the complexity of the joint, the fact that there are two joints with one bone, that there are teeth in there, and that it is an area of growth and development; these are all important points. These considerations make the whole problem of treating the TMJ extremely difficult. The importance of diagnosing and treating developmental deformities early, such as unilateral hyperplasia, cannot be overstressed. There is a little bit of confusion in the literature between subluxation and chronic dislocation, as Dr. *Laskin* stated. Another confusion to consider is the difference between being locked open or locked closed. Dr. *Laskin* was talking about the patient who is locked open. I don't really see that many patients who are locked open but I see a lot who are locked closed. He made a very good point that it is really the articular tubercle which is seen on a transcranial film. The procedure that is so often described as an eminectomy should probably be called a tuberculectomy. I think as far as the sclerosing agents go, this is probably where the answer lies for chronic recurrent dislocation. In addition, I think using fluoroscopy can help direct an injection into the ligament rather than into the joint space. Regarding Dr. *Laskin's* talk on ankylosis, I think the point was well made that surgery should maintain the height of the ramus by using interpositional material such as Silastic or vitalium. Dr. *Laskin* mentioned that functional rehabilitation is extremely important after surgery. Concerning rheumatoid arthritis, there are four different phases of rheumatoid arthritis and I think that the first stages are normally quite painful while the latter stages are not very painful. I also believe that the conservative medical management of these people is certainly in line. With degenerative arthritis, a certain number of patients can be asymptomatic. In degenerative arthritis the three different types of remodeling are regressive, progressive, and peripheral. I don't agree with Dr. *Laskin* that painful degenerative arthritis is caused from MPD syndrome. I believe that painful degenerative arthritis is strictly caused by a dislocation of the disc. As far as the treatment of degenerative joint disease I agree 100% that a meniscectomy and a condylectomy are bad. A conservative arthroplasty is an excellent procedure and I also believe that it is quite possible to reposition the articular disc. I feel we have a good diagnostic procedure which, with arthrograms, can very well determine if the disc is out of place or not. I agree it is extremely important, as Dr. *Laskin* said, to establish a diagnosis before surgery. Most important, every effort should be made to treat the patient "conservatively" before we do surgery.

One final comment about the majority of patients who present with the collection of symptoms that Dr. *Laskin* has described as the MPD syndrome. I divide things a little bit differently, and put my patients into three categories. The first is what I call nonarticular problems, which mimic temporomandibular joint pathology. There are a myriad of pathologies that can produce either pain, dysfunction or a combination of the two, but these are, as stated, nonarticular problems and essentially never involve the temporomandibular joint. My second category is the true pathologic conditions which involve the temporomandibular joint. The third group I categorize as MPD patients, whose problems do not involve the joint initially but can secondarily involve the joint.

*Dr. Solberg*

Dr. *Laskin*, where do the findings of disc displacement that Dr. *Blaschke* has pointed out through arthrography fit into your classification?

*Dr. Laskin*

Well, I have had difficulty classifying them, but I suppose they would come under early degenerative arthritis.

*Dr. Solberg*

Would this then be a secondary degenerative arthritis rather than a primary?

*Dr. Laskin*

I reserve the term primary for the group of asymptomatic, usually older patients. If you happen to take radiographs on these patients, you are going to see something wrong with the joint, but clinically you wouldn't notice anything.

*Dr. Moffett*

I just wanted to make some observations about the views that were communicated. First, I would challenge the statement that the TMJ is as unique as Dr. *Laskin* tends to portray it in comparison to other joints. I don't think that this is, in fact, true; and I think that as long as that view prevails among those who do TMJ surgery the state of the art will not take advantage of what has been learned in the management of other articulations of the body. I think the TMJ shows the same kinds of responses as other articulations do. I will agree there are developmental differences, and that because of its location it is an extremely difficult joint to approach surgically and to manipulate successfully. I believe this latter fact has been given so much attention in the training of an individual who is going to operate in this area, that it is difficult for him to learn what should be done when he has successfully entered the joint. I think oral surgery is an area where the training of the individual is not characterized by a graduate program, but more by a residency. An oral surgery resident has to learn the techniques and spend so much time and energy on that that there is not much opportunity left over for developing biologic insight or improving this state of the art. The final comment I would have to make is that in spite of the fact that I have spent my whole career trying to learn something about the TMJ, I have not yet had an opportunity to talk to a group of surgeons about what I have learned concerning this joint! I hope before I die I will have such an opportunity, but I must say, the people who operate on this joint seem to have a wall around them. There is some kind of overemphasis on technique which makes the surgical specialist think that he has nothing to learn from individuals who don't go in and operate on the joint.

Dr. *Mahan*

One comment on some data in *Toller*'s paper in 1973 where he had followed 130 degenerative arthritis jaw joint patients over 17 years, and reported 44% of these patients had what he called TMJ pain dysfunction or MPD syndrome. There was a high incidence in his paper of a previous history of MPD in the cases that he classified as degenerative arthritis. I also have one quick question. Dr. *Laskin*, you pointed out that growth arrest coincides with antegional notching and I ask is the reverse true. Does antegional notching mean growth arrest?

*Dr. Laskin*

I have always believed when you have exaggeration of the antegonial notch it indicates that there is some growth deficiency.

# VII. Temporomandibular Joint Changes Related to Dental Occlusion

by Tore Hansson

Temporomandibular joints and muscles, like all other joints and muscles of the body, can be affected by a variety of diseases. Presumably, the most common group, including those occurring in the teeth and periodontium, are diseases due to loading.[1] Biomechanical loading during function and parafunction plays a dominant role in the initiation and development of these tissue changes. I will focus today on temporomandibular joint (TMJ) changes related to biomechanical loading and dental occlusion, but first some words about the multifactorial etiology behind TMJ diseases. (Fig. 1).

*Local factors* are capable of creating adverse loading resulting in irritating microtrauma to the joint tissues. These factors might often be changes in the functional anatomy of occlusion. While results from different investigations support the theory that extensive tooth loss predisposes one to TMJ disease, more limited occlusal interferences also seem to be important. Several studies have shown that *psychic factors* increase muscle tension resulting in bruxism with heavy loading. *Somatic systemic factors* can be contributory by influencing the ability of the joint tissues to resist an increased biomechanical load. The ability of the articulating tissues of the joints to resist pressure and wear and tear depends largely on their physical and chemical properties. A number of factors: genetic, endocrine, metabolic and vascular, which may vary with sex and age, can alter these properties of the joint tissues and joint fluids and therefore influence the development and progress of arthrosis. The quality of cartilage, for example, is dependent on the structure of the proteoglycans which are in high concentration there. The high content of aggregates of proteoglycans increases the tolerance of the joint to pressure due to the electrostatically repulsive glucosaminoglycans. Elasticity (chondroitinsulphate) diminishes in older and degenerative cartilage, because of degeneration of the different "arms" of the proteoglycan chains.[2] However, we have to keep in mind that the etiology of the TMJ-diseases seems very often to be multifactorial with contributing factors from **all** the three groups. (For literature review, see *Carlsson, Kopp* and *Oberg,* 1979.)[3]

The temporomandibular joint ceases to grow at about 20 years of age, but throughout the rest of life the soft and hard tissue layers of the articulating components continue to undergo structural changes, i. e., remodeling.[4] Remodeling, progressive or regressive in nature, is so slight under optimal conditions that joint form appropriate to smooth function is maintained. In healthy TMJs, the articulating surfaces are gently rounded and smooth even in older age groups. The following tissue layers are found in both the condyle and the temporal component: 1) connective tissue lining, which forms the articular surface, 2) undifferentiated

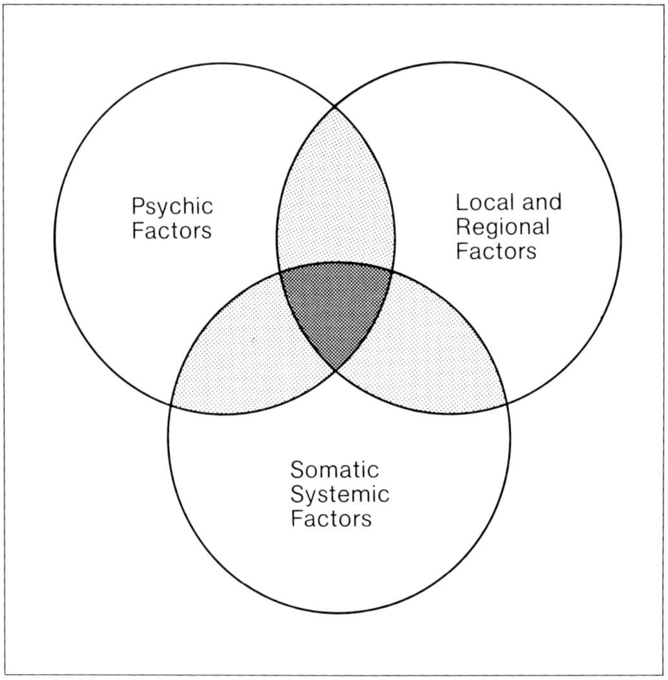


Fig. 1 Main etiological factors of diseases due to loading.

mesenchyme, the proliferating layer, 3) transitional layer, which is indistinct, 4) fibrous cartilage, 5) compact bone and 6) spongy bone. The soft tissue layers (the connective tissue lining, the undifferentiated mesenchyme and most of the fibrous cartilage) form the covering of the hard tissues of the condyle and the temporal component. In both the components the soft tissue covering varies considerably in thickness, differing with anatomic location.

When the soft tissue layers of 48 TMJ autopsy specimens without any gross sign of diseases were measured, the mean value of the soft tissue thickness was highest postero-inferiorly on the articular tubercle ~ 0.5 mm and lowest in the roof of fossa ~ 0.1 mm. In the condyle the soft tissues were thickest superiorly ~ 0.5 mm and supero-anteriorly ~ 0.4 mm and thinnest posteriorly ~ 0.25 mm.[5]

The differences in thickness in adult joints reflect variations in biomechanical loading in the joint. This depends chiefly on the loading stimulating a proliferative response in the undifferentiated mesenchyme. A fairly thick cartilage develops postero-inferiorly on the articular tubercle, but no cartilage formation appears in the roof of the fossa. This corresponds to the areas normally exposed to maximum and minimum pressures, respectively. The undifferentiated mesenchyme may be utilized for cartilage formation to such an extent that it disappears as a continous tissue layer.[6]

The disc is passively adapted to the contours of the temporal component and of the condyle due to its form and makeup of collagenous fibrous connective tissue.[7,8] In healthy joints the disc is thinnest in the middle dense parts, mean value ~ 1 mm.[5]

The posterior loose part of the disc, which is

very rich in vessels and nerve endings, must be more throughly investigated in the future. We know little about patho-anatomical changes there. But we know that many patients suffer from different forms of pain and movement disturbances of the lower jaw without any radiographic signs of disease. The joints might be tender to palpation, very often both laterally and posteriorly, and exhibit reduced condylar mobility, with pain during passive movements to eccentric jaw positions. Repeated overload on the joint capsule, and loose part of the disc, as well as on the attachment of the lateral pterygoid muscle can cause reactions of inflammation, i.e., synovitis and edema. Findings of thrombosis and thrombophlebitis in this area have also been ascribed to irritating microtraumata.[9,10] Arthritis microtraumatica, an inflammatory reaction in the capsule, loose peripheral parts of the disc and the insertion of the lateral pterygoid muscle due to repeated compression and traction during function and parafunction, is probably the most common disease of the temporomandibular joint and is very often in combination with other diseases due to loading. Unstable occlusion must be regarded as an etiologic factor behind TMJ arthritis microtraumatica, but the opinions about the interferences as etiologic factors for TMJ-changes are controversial.[11] Many authors agree, however that disharmony of occlusion can disturb the stomatognathic function. That occlusal instability leads to neuromuscular and at least functional joint disturbances seems to be a common opinion among many clinicians, and many patients are treated for different symptoms by occlusal adjustment. Several investigators have found that occlusal interferences are more frequent among patients than in non-patient groups.[12, 13, 14]

In an experimental study on 8 healthy students, *Randow* et al. (1976)[15] inserted an occlusal interference (gold inlay) on the path of closure of the mandible. The inlay was placed in one of the mandibular first molars (0.25 mm in height). An immediate disturbance of the muscular pattern was registered electromyographically. During the time (14 days) of the experiment, dysfunctional symptoms were noted in all but one of the subjects. One student suffered from TMJ-problems for a considerable time after the experiment.

We investigated thirty healthy students for tenderness of the TMJ and of the masseter, temporal and lateral pterygoid muscles. Interferences were checked before the electromyographical investigation. About half of them had an occlusal adjustment performed and immediately thereafter a new electromyogram was run. (Fig. 2). The occlusal adjustment caused an immediate response in the musculature producing better coordination of muscle function in the subjects who had marked interferences between retruded contact position (RCP) and intercuspal position (ICP).

*Solberg* and coworkers (1979)[16] concluded from their epidemiological study on 739 UCLA students that asymmetry in the slide from RCP to ICP appeared to be associated with dysfunctional signs, but the length of the slide was not associated with the signs. Tenderness of the TMJs was also associated with asymmetrical slides from RCP. Reducing or eliminating interferences between RCP and ICP in patients has often been looked upon as clinical opinion without scientific proof. The results from the UCLA investigation[16] and from different experimental studies indicate that the interferences between RCP and ICP are important factors in the etiology of TMJ-diseases. Therefore, I would suggest that it is a professional duty to eliminate those interferences in the treatment setting.

Remodeling processes may be so advanced that they produce deviations in form (DIF) of

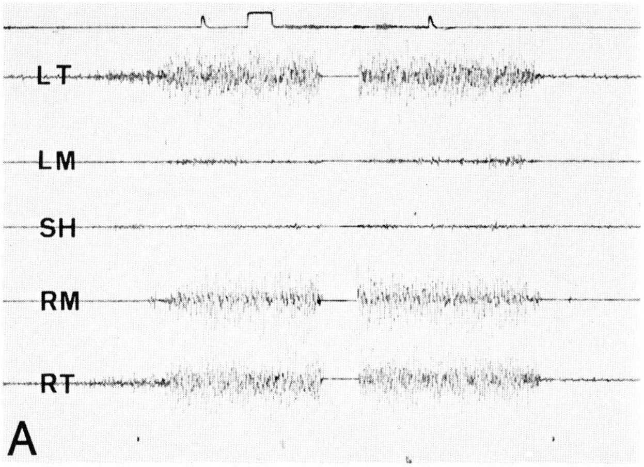


Fig. 2 Subject with left side TMJ – and muscular tenderness to palpation. Marked interference between RCP and ICP on left side first molars.

A. Extremely reduced activity in left masseter muscle (LM) in ICP before occlusal adjustment.

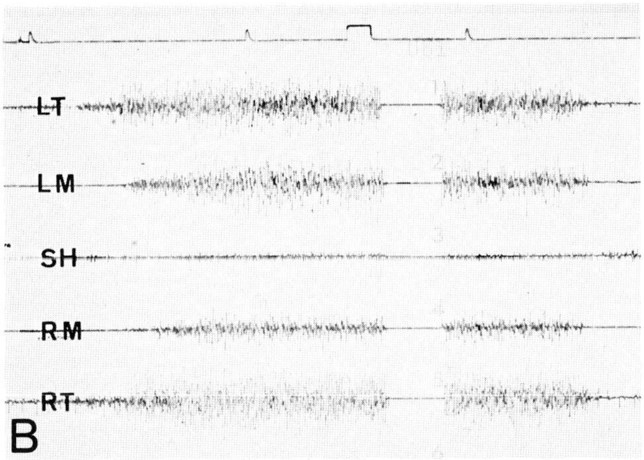


B. Immediate response in left masseter muscle (LM) in ICP after occlusal adjustment.

the articulating components which interfere with joint function.[4,17] Eventually the changes may progress to pathological conditions, such as arthrosis, representing destruction of the articulating surface layer. (Fig. 3).

In Swedish autopsy material, *Öberg* and coworkers found that about half of the 102 adult TMJs either showed arthrotic lesions or had deviations in form (DIF) of such a character and degree that they could be expected to cause irregular joint movements. Marked deviations in form were found in almost one-fourth (24) of the joints.[17, 18] They were already common in the 20—40 year age groups. (Table 1). The deviations in form were predominantly localized to the lateral part of the joint and the frequency was higher in the condyle than in the temporal component. In autopsy material from the Los Angeles County Morgue consisting of young temporomandibular joints between 17 and 37 years of age, *Hansson* et al. (1979)[19] found that 26 out of 30 joints revealed DIF in one or more components. The deviations in form were also located in the lateral and central parts of the joint.

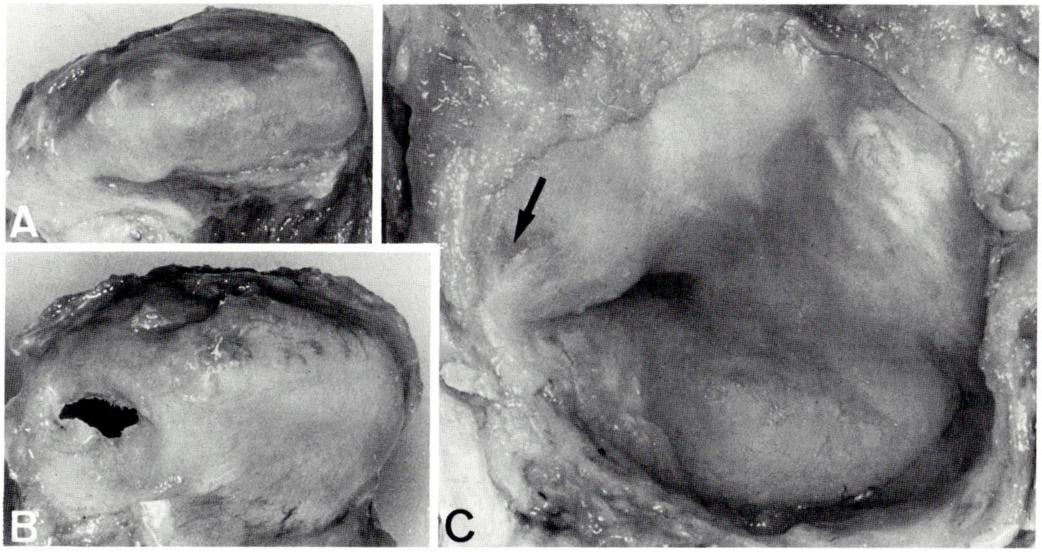


Fig. 3 Deviations in form (DIF) in the lateral parts of the condyle (A) and of the temporal component (C) have produced a perforation of the disc (B). This arthrotic lesion is situated just opposite to the elevations of the other two components. On the articular tubercle of the temporal component (C) is also seen a shallow arthrotic lesion (arrow). (From *Öberg, Carlsson* and *Fajers*, 1971).

The deviations in form (DIF) are the result of the sum of progressive and regressive remodeling in the tissue layers. *Bean, Omnell* and *Öberg* (1977)[20] concluded, after removal of the soft tissues from 20 TMJs, that DIF are due not only to remodeling of hard tissue, but also to a large extent to variations of thickness of soft tissue. In 22 TMJs with DIF, *Hansson* and *Nordstrom* (1977)[6] measured the soft tissue layers and also found that these layers played an important role in the development of DIF. In the joints with DIF the soft tissue covering was generally thicker than in the healthy joints, especially in the lateral part of the joint. The increase in thickness was related to the cartilage, which (as was pointed out earlier) develops from the undifferentiated mesenchyme. This proliferating layer had thereby been utilized to such an extent that it remained to a significantly lesser degree in the joints with DIF. Probably, the reactive capacity of the joint components had also been lowered through the reduction

**Table I** Classification of the adult joints

| | number of joints | | 20-39 years | 40-93 years |
|---|---|---|---|---|
| Normal joints | 53 | | 14 | 39 |
| Joints with only deviations in form | 24 | | 8 | 16 |
| Joints with only arthrosis | 3 | 48 | 1 | 2 |
| Joints with both deviations in form and arthrosis | 21 | | 0 | 21 |
| Malformed joint | 1 | | 1 | 0 |
| Total joints | 102 | | 24 | 78 |

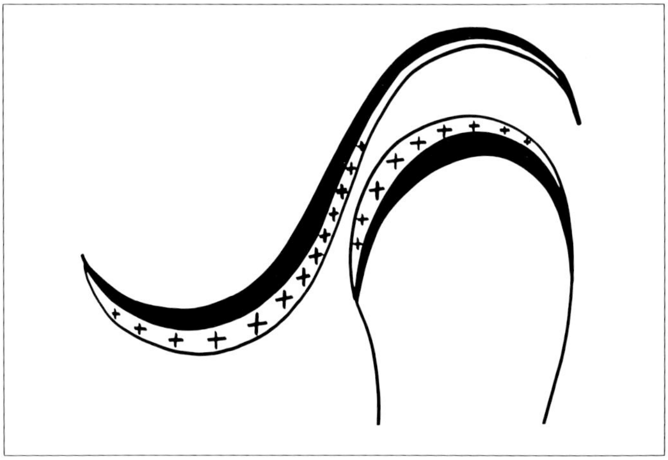

Fig. 4 Localization of the dimensional changes of the soft tissue thickness between healthy TMJ-s and TMJ-s with deviations in form. The disc is passively adapted to the deviations in form of the condyle and of the temporal component.

of this layer. There was significantly more of the undifferentiated mesenchyme in the condyle than in the temporal component, indicating a higher remodeling capacity in the condyle.

The thickness of the fibrous connective tissue lining (the surface layer) did not differ between the joints with DIF and healthy joints. Experimental studies on laboratory animals have also shown that the surface layer is only passively involved in the changes in form.[7,8] Thus, it is the reactive capacity of undifferentiated mesenchyme which is mainly responsible for the dimensional changes in the soft tissue covering. (Fig. 4)

In general, the disc was thinner laterally in the joints with DIF than in the healthy joints. Obviously, this was due to the passive adaptation to the DIF in the other components and to the pressure loading.

In the Swedish autopsy material,[17, 18] joints with DIF seem be common in young people, while arthrotic joints were found in only 4% in the age group of 20—39 years. In the groups over 39 years, arthrosis was observed in 30% of the specimens. Only three of the arthrotic joints did not reveal remarkable DIF. It seems that after 40 years of age many of the untreated joints with DIF can progress to arthrosis. Of 24 arthrotic joints, 20 had local injuries and 4 had extensive lesions. The lesions were generally found in the lateral portions of the joints, as were the DIF. In 15 of the joints the injuries were laterally located, in 5 they were central, but in none was any lesion seen in the most medial part. The lesions were more common in the disc and the temporal component than in the condyle, (whereas deviations in form were most common in the condyle). Arthrosis was seen in the disc in 17, in the temporal component in 14 and in the condyle in only one out of the 20 joints with local arthrotic injuries. In the temporal component the local arthrotic lesion is most common in the fossa and on the posterior slope of the articular tubercle. The frequency is highest in the lateral wall of the fossa and laterally on the posterior slope of the tubercle. In the disc and in the condyle the lesions are seen in juxtaposed areas. When there is DIF on the condyle and the temporal component, the injury first affects the disc or the temporal component. In thin areas, the

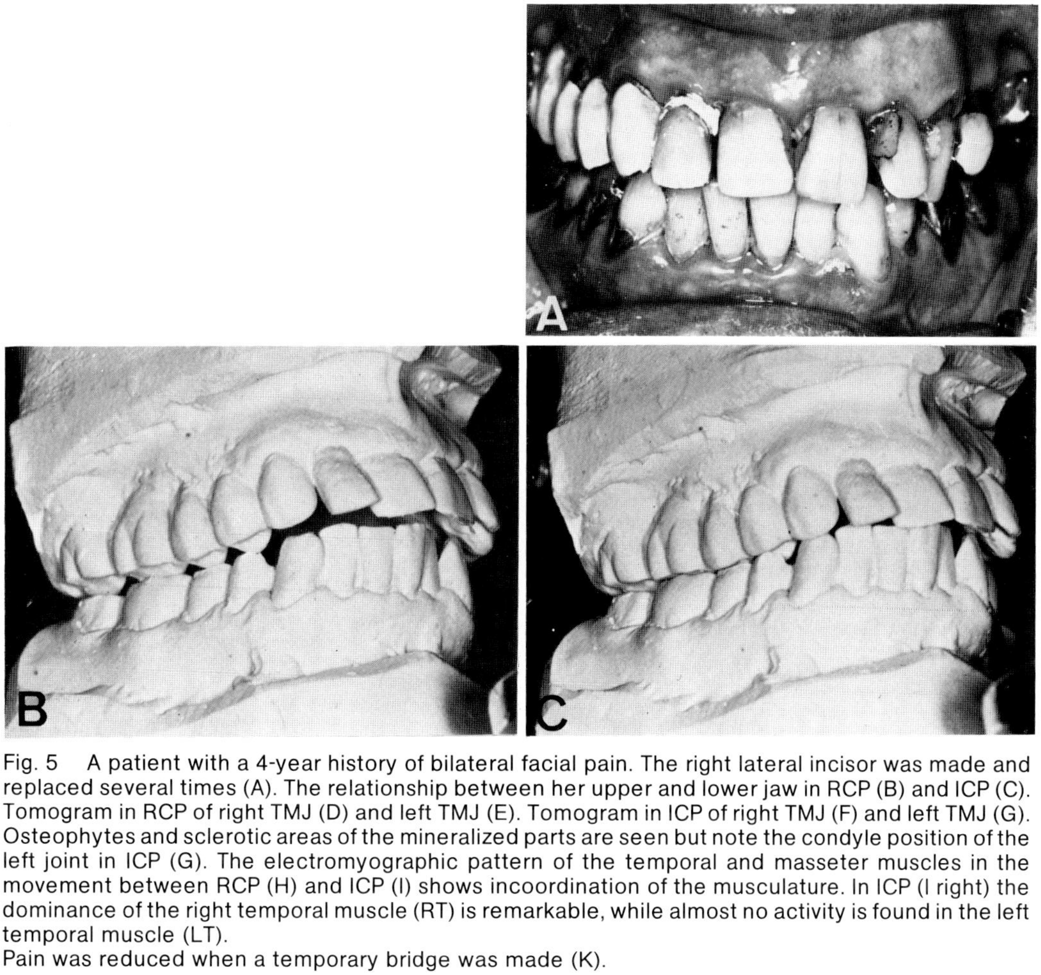


Fig. 5 A patient with a 4-year history of bilateral facial pain. The right lateral incisor was made and replaced several times (A). The relationship between her upper and lower jaw in RCP (B) and ICP (C). Tomogram in RCP of right TMJ (D) and left TMJ (E). Tomogram in ICP of right TMJ (F) and left TMJ (G). Osteophytes and sclerotic areas of the mineralized parts are seen but note the condyle position of the left joint in ICP (G). The electromyographic pattern of the temporal and masseter muscles in the movement between RCP (H) and ICP (I) shows incoordination of the musculature. In ICP (I right) the dominance of the right temporal muscle (RT) is remarkable, while almost no activity is found in the left temporal muscle (LT).
Pain was reduced when a temporary bridge was made (K).

disc is often perforated. The articulating surface of the condyle is damaged last and, most often, not at all.

The difference in the frequency of DIF and arthrosis in the three articulating joint components seems to be related to *differences in their reactive capacity to biomechanical loading.* This is due to variations in histologic construction and appears to be particularly valid for the undifferentiated mesenchyme with its high reactive and remodeling capacity. There is more of this tissue in the condyle than in the temporal component.[7] No such tissue layer is present in the disc. Even in joints with DIF, more remnants of undifferentiated mesenchyme are present in the condyle than in the temporal component.[6] These differences in reactive capacity may be an explanation why such a large number of DIF of the condyle was found in the studies, while arthrotic lesions, on the other hand, were markedly fewer in the con-

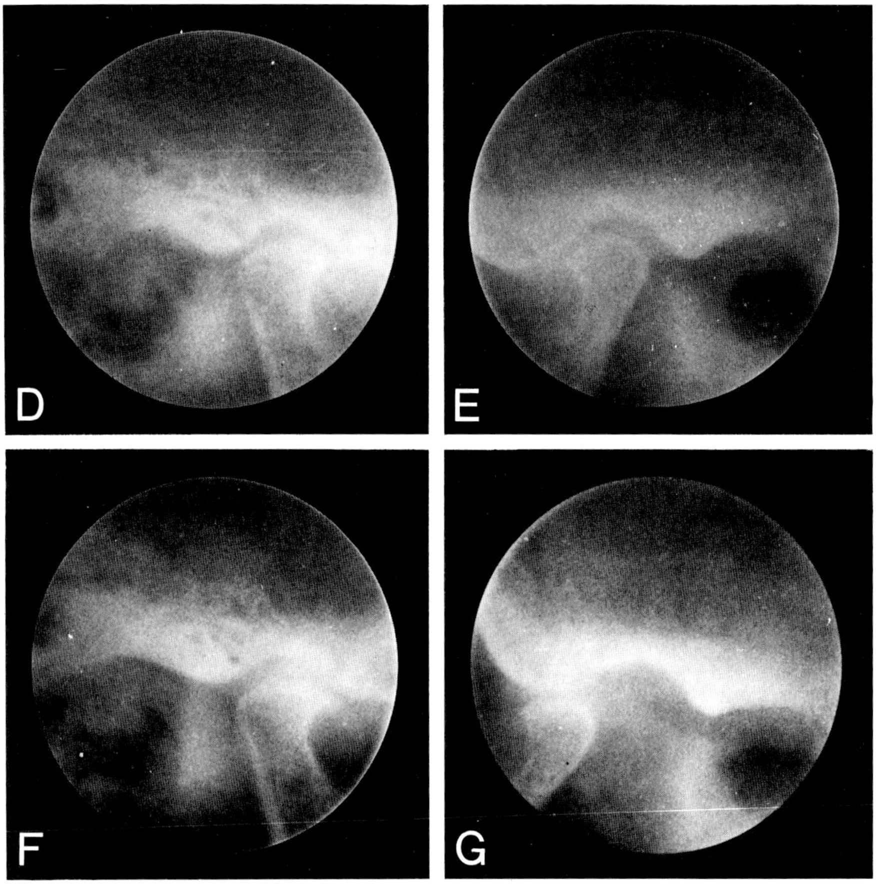


Fig. 5d–g

dyle than in the disc and in the temporal component. *The undifferentiated mesenchyme may thus be regarded as a protecting factor for the joint.*

The morphological characteristics, the localization of the DIF, and the relationship of arthrotic lesions in the articulating components, allow no serious question that biomechancial factors are significant in causing these changes. Experimental studies on laboratory animals also support the opinion that the biomechanics of the joint are of decisive importance in remodeling and in the development of arthrosis. A comparison between the temporomandibular joint and two other joints in the Swedish autopsy material also suggests that local factors are more important than systemic factors for development of arthrotic lesions.[21]

As for the biomechanical factors, *Öberg* and coworkers (1971)[18] showed that extensive loss of teeth predisposes to changes in the functional loading of the TMJ, which may then lead to deviation in form and arthrosis. *Kopp* (1977)[22] concluded that molar loss plays a role in the etiology of TMJ-arthrosis when he compared (19) patients with TMJ palpatory tenderness to other patients with mandibular dysfunction. Last year, forty-four adult skulls from the 11th century were

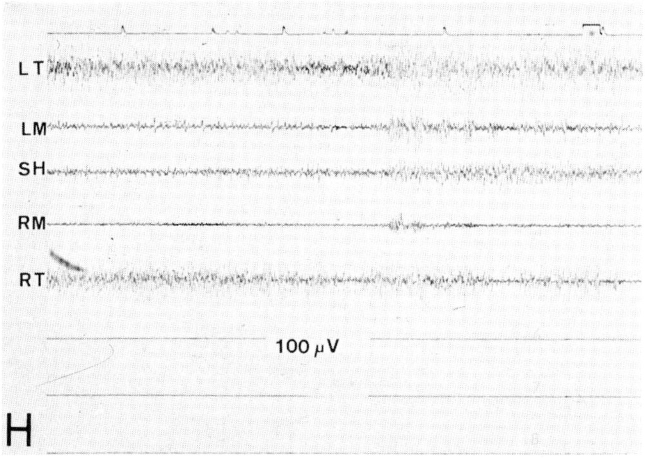


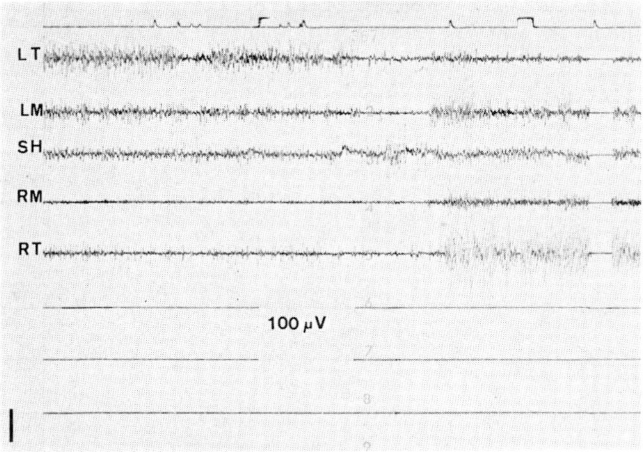


Fig. 5h–i

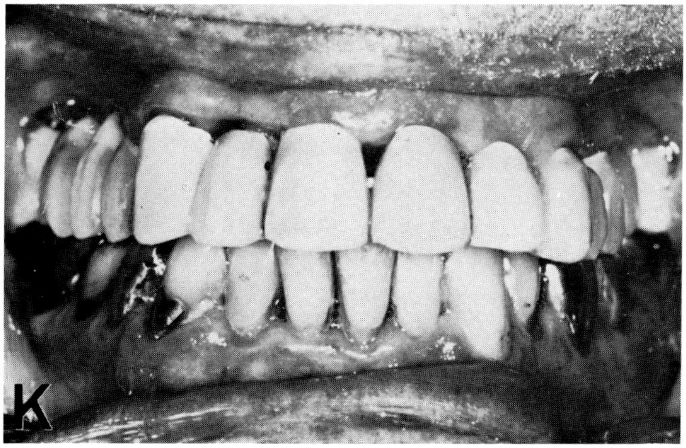


Fig. 5k

examined for TMJ-changes by *Bergman* and *Hansson*[23]. Loss of premolars and molars bilaterally were correlated to changes in form of the condyle and to destruction of hard tissue on the inferior part of the articular tubercle.

Another possible factor contributing to the changes might be abrasion. After an investigation on 100 skulls, *Mongini* (1975)[24] concluded that abrasion influenced changes in condyle shape due to bone remodeling. In our skull material,[23] changes in form and destruction of hard tissues were correlated with abrasion even on the temporal component. The areas affected were the same as those where the thickened soft tissue was found in the autopsy material. *Wedel, Carlsson* and *Sagne* (1978)[25] had the same findings in another sample of skull material, 48 crania, from the south of Sweden.

In summary, changes in biomechanical loading of the temporomandibular joint may cause remodeling of progressive and regressive nature in the soft and hard tissue layers of the joint components. Even in young adults, the remodeling is often so advanced that it causes DIF of the articulating components and creates a mechanical impediment to joint function. The functional disturbances may further alter and intensify functional loading of joint tissue and, untreated, gradually lead to arthrosis. (Fig. 5)

Prophylactic dental methods are therefore indicated not only to prevent further loss of teeth, but also to preserve the health of TMJ-tissues. Simple dental methods to improve the occlusion are often sufficient to stop or inhibit the development of arthrosis.

Dentists are the only therapists who are capable of preventing future TMJ pain caused by unstable occlusion.

## References


1. *Carlsson, G. E., Öberg, T.*
Remodelling of the temporomandibular joint. Chapter 5. In Temporomandibular Joint, Function and Dysfunction. Eds. George A. Zarb & Gunnar E. Carlsson, Munksgaard, Copenhagen. The C. V. Mosby Company, St. Louis, Missouri, 1979

2. *Ineroth, S., Heinegård, D., Andell, L., Olson, S. E.*
Articular cartilage proteoglycans in aging and osteoarthritis. Biochem. J. In press

3. *Carlsson, G. E., Kopp, S., Öberg, T.*
Arthritis and allied diseases of the temporomandibular joint. Chapter 10. In Temporomandibular Joint, Function and Dysfunction.
Eds. George A. Zarb & Gunner E. Carlsson. Munksgaard, Copenhagen. The C. V. Mosby Company, St. Louis, Missouri, 1979

4. *Hansson, T.*
Temporomandibular joint changes, occurence and development. Thesis. University of Lund, Malmö, Sweden. 1977

5. *Hansson, T., Öberg, T., Carlsson, G. E., Kopp, S.*
Thickness of the soft tissue layers and the articular disc in the temporomandibular joint.
Acta Odontol. Scand. 35:77—83. 1977

6. *Hansson, T., Nordström, B.*
Thickness of the soft tissue layers and articular disc in temporomandibular joints with deviations in form.
Acta Odontol. Scand. 35:281—288. 1977

7. *Öberg, T.*
Morphology, growth and matrix formation in the mandibular joint of the guinea pig. Diss. Trans. Royal Schools of Dentistry, Stockholm/Umeå, No. 10. 1964

8. *Blackwood, H. J. J.*
Cellular remodelling in articular tissue. J. Dent. Res. 45:480—489. 1966

9. *Griffin, C. J., Sharpe, C. J.*
Pressure atrophy of the human temporomandibular meniscus associated with thrombosis of an articular branch of the pterygoid arteries.
Austr. Dent. J. 6:32—34. 1961

10. *Griffin, C. J., Barnett, A. V.*
A preliminary report on plastic thrombophlebitis in the pterygocondylar area and its clinical and pathological significance.
Oral Surg. II:1323—1336. 1958

11. *Carlsson, G. E.*
The consequences of occlusal interferences. Chapter 15. In Prosthodontic Treatment for Partially Edentulous Patients. Eds. Zarb, G. A., Bergman, B., Clayton, J. A. and McKay, H. F. C. V. Mosby Company St. Louis, Missouri. 1978

12. *Agerberg, G., Carlsson, G. E., Ericson, S., Lundberg, M., Öberg, T.* Funktionsrubbningar i tuggapparaten. En bettfysiologisk, röntgenologisk och serologisk undersökning. Svensk Tandläk. Tidskrift 62:1192—1211. 1970

13. *Rosell, C. G., Öberg, T.* Remissorsak „Käkledsbesvär". Undersökning av ett patientmaterial vid en centraltandpoliklinik. Tandläkaretidningen 67:941—950. 1975

14. *Carlsson, G. E., Magnusson, T., Wedel, A.* Patientmaterialet vid en bettfysiologisk avdelning. Swed. Dent. J. 69:115—121. 1976

15. *Randow, K., Carlsson, G. E., Edlund, J., Öberg, T.* The effect of an occlusal interference on the masticatory system. An experimental investigation. Odont. Revy 27:245—256. 1976

16. *Solberg, W. K., Woo, M. W., Houston, J. B.* Prevalence of mandibular dysfunction in young adults. JADA 98:25—34. 1979

17. *Hansson, T. Öberg, T.* Arthrosis and deviation in form in the temporomandibular joint. A macroscopic study on a human autopsy material. Acta Odontol. Scand. 35:167—174. 1977

18. *Öberg, T., Carlsson, G. E., Fajers, C. M.* The temporomandibular joint. A morphologic study on a human autopsy material. Acta Odontol. Scand. 29:349—384. 1971

19. *Hansson, T., Öberg, T., Solberg, W. K., Penn, M. K.* Anatomic study of the TMJs of young adults. A pilot investigation. J. Pros. Dent. 41:556—560. 1979

20. *Bean, L. R., Omnell, K. Å., Öberg, T.* Comparisons between radiologic observations and macroscopic tissue changes in temporomandibular joints. Dentomaxillofac. Radiol. 6:90—106. 1977

21. *Kopp, S., Carlsson, G. E., Hansson, T., Öberg, T.* Degenerative disease in the temporomandibular, metatarsophalangeal and sternoclavicular joints. An autopsy study. Acta Odontol. Scand. 34:23—32. 1976

22. *Kopp, S.* Clinical findings in temporomandibular joint osteoarthrosis. Scand. J. Dent. Res. 85:434, 1977.

23. *Bergman, L. E., Hansson, T.* TMJ-changes in an archaeo-osteological material. Swed. Dent. J., 3:149-155, 1979.

24. *Mongini, F.* Dental abrasion as a factor in remodelling of the mandibular condyle. Acta Anat. 92:292—300. 1975

25. *Wedel, A., Carlsson, G. E., Sagne, S.* Temporomandibular joint morphology in a medieval skull material. Swed. Dent. J. 2:177—187. 1978


# Discussion

Discussant: Benjamin Moffett

*Dr. Moffett*

I will try to contribute what insights I can, as a nonclinician, to the development of clinical arts related to the management of occlusion. First of all, I would like to define occlusion in a way which seems to be logical or useful from my point of view — and my definition changes with time. At the present time, if I had to define occlusion, I would say it is the shifting equilibrium between form and function that is influenced by every event of morphologic, physiologic, pathologic, psychologic or dental significance for this part of the body. In that regard, I think it is obvious that we are dealing with a multifactorial problem.

I remember how I once struggled with one of my orthodontic colleagues to attempt to demonstrate a relationship between the form of the dentition, (occlusal surfaces of the teeth) and the form of a temporomandibular joint in dry skulls using a single factorial approach. Before we had access to computer methodology and multifactorial analysis, we could only pull out one variable at a time and test for its significance in what was really a multifactorial situation. Every investigator at that time, including myself, ended up with statistically insignificant results, because the tools were not adequate to analyze such a multifactorial problem. I think that if the investigator wishes to succeed in showing a relationship between the TMJ and the dental occlusion, he has to take advantage of an important advance in methodology-computer analysis.

Another problem to be faced is our tendency to associate TMJ changes related to dental occlusion with morphologic changes. If we are going to practice a biologic approach to the management of clinical problems in dentistry, we must simultaneously monitor changes in function, as well as changes in form. I am working now in a clinical discipline (orthodontics) which historically has concluded that only changes in skeletal form and occlusal form have to be documented, and that if there are changes in occlusal function happening at the same time, they are unimportant and need not be documented. New approaches must include electromyography. I think this is such a complex problem, that these relationships can only be documented adequately by a team approach. For instance, besides monitoring muscle function through EMG activity, I think we have to use the techniques of jaw tracking being developed at my school and at the dental school in Vancouver, where we simultaneously compare changes in EMG activity with changes in jaw function, for instance, in individuals with different kinds of occlusion, or in individuals who have had therapeutic occlusal alterations. If we can get all of these multifactorial aspects documented at the same time, a task which is becoming more and more feasible, then I think that we will be able to show effectively that there is a true relationship between changes in the function, movements and form of the TMJ and the changes in form and function of occlusion. I think it is a tremendously difficult problem and it is going to require very close cooperation between nonclinicians and clinicians. My plea is to give individuals who are nonclinicians, and who are interested in these problems, an opportunity to participate in dialogues with clinical specialists who are trying to cope with these tremendous problems. If my function as a professional scientist in dentistry (I left the discipline of anatomy two decades ago) requires me to be self-critical, then I hope you will respond to that self-criticism in a constructive way and not look on it as an adversarial relationship. I have indicated earlier that I think the clinician and the laboratory worker are both researchers, and in trying to find out what is good methodology for colleagues like Dr. *Hansson* and me to follow, we need to practice a kind of thinking in our research and our documentation that is both logical and self-critical. If I make self-critical comments, I do so not as an outsider looking in on dentistry but rather, as a colleague trying to share information that might be of help to you. I commend the efforts of Dr. *Hansson* and his colleagues, and I offer these suggestions as an aid to further success in the documentation that he is carrying out which is already, very successful. With the new kinds of technology and methodology in research, there are other individuals,Dr. *Hansson*, who can help you and me attempt to provide this kind of documentation. Now it has been said by some of our colleagues in dentistry that we have not experimentally demonstrated the significance of occlusion in TMJ function and dysfunction. I beg to differ with that. In fact, I think that none of us have adequately established a satisfactory experimental basis for the concepts that we have in any of the various clinical specialities in dentistry. With these comments, as a response to your commendable efforts, I would open the discussion to other members of the panel and the floor.

*Dr. Solberg*

Dr. *Hansson,* I would like to ask you to clarify one point concerning the two interesting cases where you found what appeared to me to be evidence of abnormally retruded condyles. The condyles were more or less retruded relative to the mandibular fossas. You put a splint on these patients that was rather thick and you showed post-treatment views that appeared to show that the condyles had moved to a more concentric position. Can you comment further on why that happened or what you did to make that occur? You obviously were not repositioning the condyles forward by jumping the bite.

*Dr. Hansson*

We have seen many times that if we make the splints about 3 mm in thickness and in a retruded position, as we usually do, our radiographic surveys often show a distraction of the condyle in the joint. There is no special art for manipulating the joint position. This is just a clinical result, and we have some thoughts on how it could have happened. There might also be internal changes in the temporomandibular joint that you can alter, and it might be that thickening of the soft tissue is so local in the beginning, that just a little rotation could alter some positions.

*Dr. Solberg*

Thank you. I would like to ask Dr. *Öberg* if he has any comments relative to Dr. *Hansson's* discussion or, in fact, to any previous discussion.

*Dr. Öberg*

Yes. After the work of Tore Hansson, we have tried in Malmö to look at the joint, the muscles and also the teeth, all together, and I think that the loading diseases may appear at the same time in each of these tissues. We may, perhaps, have the first clinical symptoms from the muscles, but I think you have simultaneous remodeling changes in the temporomandibular joint, in both the soft and hard tissue layers of the joint which may then develop into true pathological changes. So in my opinion, the changes are going on in parallel. It is not an either/or; it is a both/and. It is a matter of morphofunctional harmony about which Dr. *Krogh-Poulsen* has so often spoken. I think also that biochemical factors, such as proteoglycans, are subjects of very interesting research now in the chemical laboratories. For example, in the medical school in Lund, Sweden they have shown that there is degradation of proteoglycans with age. So age is a factor, but not a decisive or predominant one. They have also done experiments on greyhounds, where they operated on the pelvis, altering the mechanical situation in the joint without going into it. At first, you have a degradation of these aggregates of proteoglycans and then the arthrotic lesion develops.

*Dr. Mahan*

In your corrosive specimens you destroyed or removed the soft tissues, where did the corrosion stop? Did you just remove the collagen or did you remove the cartilage? Did it stop at the cartilage or at the bone?

*Dr. Hansson*

That was the study made by *Bean, Omnell* and *Öberg* (1977).

*Dr. Öberg*

All the soft tissue was removed, but the most inferior part of the cartilage is mineralized so there was compact bone and mineralized cartilage on the surface. Two to four cell rows of the cartilage are mineralized. So the soft tissue is anything else on the top.

*Dr. Mahan*

In studies of the hip joint in rabbits, it has been found that if you impact load the joint, that is, drive the femur into the acetabulum with one stroke a second for an hour a day, after 30 days you get the loss of the acid mucopolysaccharides. You show this phenomenon with age and we see it with microtrauma of impact loading the hip where you have a good deal more cartilage. You differentiate between arthrosis and deviation in form. Could you clarify that again? You have deviation in form which leads to arthrosis, and what is your differentiation? You were critical of *Toller's* concept of TMJ arthrosis (1973) and that is an issue I would like to straighten out in my mind.

*Dr. Hansson*

The deviation in form is a deviation from the normally rounded contour of the articular surface due to remodeling in hard and soft tissues. The arthrosis is a noninflammatory joint disease characterized by wear and tear of the articulating joint surface and by simultaneous remodeling of the underlying hard tissues.

*Dr. Mahan*

You mean that the deviation in form didn't involve the remodeling of the bone underneath?

*Dr. Öberg*

Bony changes go on in parallel, too. You will never have changes in the soft tissue without changes in the hard tissue. They are running parallel, but you can have progressive or regressive remodeling of the hard tissue, and you have erosive changes which you can see in the tomograms. If it is an arthrosis, you must have a fibrillation and a breakdown of some part of the soft tissue layer.

*Dr. Solberg*

Dr. *Öberg,* do you consider these remodeling changes pathological if they involve the underlying bone?

*Dr. Öberg*

I think perhaps we have to say that this advanced hard tissue remodeling under the intact soft tissue is the beginning of an arthrosis, but these changes do not necessarily develop into an arthrotic lesion. If you have a perforation of the hard tissue, I think we have to look on them as pathologic. Perhaps we should develop another name for these pre-arthrotic changes. We see them very often.

*Dr. Mahan*

Would it be fair to say that you could make the distinction by saying that loss of continuity of the surface constitutes arthrosis, whereas there is not a loss of the continuity of the surface in your definition of deviation in form. Would that be correct?

*Dr. Öberg*

That is correct.

*Dr. Mahan*

So we could use the terms physiologic remodeling and pathologic remodeling. Would that also be the distinction?

*Dr. Hansson*

I think that the physiological remodeling wouldn't create marked contour differences.

*Dr. Solberg*

Dr. *Öberg,* If I understand you correctly, you are saying that there is no clear-cut distinction between physiologic remodeling and arthrosis; that there can be an intermediary condition that may or may not be completely normal.

*Dr. Öberg*

Yes, it is difficult to decide where the physiologically normal state ceases. Naturally, it is a gradual spectrum.

*Dr. Reuben Robinson* (Knoxville, Tennessee)

I would like to ask Dr. *Hansson* to elaborate on the significance of transcranial X-rays in the diagnosis and treatment of TMJ pain dysfunction. It seems to me that you are the first one at this meeting who has put any credence in the transcranial radiograph.

*Dr. Hansson*

I will trust in transcranial projections regarding structural changes but if you really want to measure the condyle position you have to take tomograms. With ordinary patients coming to the dental clinics, we can't do tomography all the time, and since I must treat the patient, I think I would trust transcranial pictures to help me.

*Dr. Donald Jones* (New Jersey)

I would like to ask you a question. I noticed that you used a predominance of maxillary occlusal splints. I wonder if you would discuss the rationale of using a maxillary versus a mandibular splint, or a full maxillary occlusal splint versus an anterior resting splint.

*Dr. Hansson*

When we educate our students, we always tell them that the main thing, as I said before, is to make a stable occlusion. We put the stabilization splint in that jaw where we have less teeth. We try to make it completely stable, so it is like a partial denture. Ten years ago we were very careful about having the splints very thin within the freeway space. Since we have worked with the electromyographic examination, parallel to the clinical manipulations of the patient, we have found that a splint of thickness two to three millimeters will get you about the same effect as if you use an upper anterior relaxation splint. With the more difficult patients we use the full arch stabilization splint.

*Dr. Yoshio Yamaguchi* (Los Angeles)

Dr. *Hansson,* after you put the splint in, what is the average time, and what criteria do you use to transfer from the splint to the more definitive crown and bridge work or other definitive occlusal therapy?

*Dr. Hannson*

As a routine, we take the patient back after one week and we readjust the splint. If it is satisfactory, we leave the splint with the patient for one month or six weeks, and if the patient is responding well, we change the splint to a permanent bridge temporarily cemented. After about three to four months, we reexamine radiographically, and then we consider permanent cementation.

# VIII. Diagnosis and Treatment of Internal Derangements of the Articular Disc and Mandibular Condyle

by William McCarty

## Introduction

The material presented here primarily represents the concepts of Dr. *William B. Farrar* of Montgomery, Alabama, who has worked with temporomandibular joint patients for the past 20 years. Bill Farrar recognized the problem with the displaced disc many years ago and has developed a method of diagnosis and treatment, incorporating a team approach of occlusal jaw repositioning, restorative dentistry, orthodontics and surgery. Credit must also be given Dr. *Clyde Wilkes* of Minneapolis, Minnesota for his pioneering work in arthrography.

This material is based on the examination and treatment of over 4000 TMJ patients, of which over 350 were treated surgically. The conclusions reached have been based on measurable diagnostic studies which can be reproduced by any interested dentist, if he is but willing to take the time.

During the past several years the dental profession has shown an increased interest in temporomandibular joint (TMJ) dysfunction and pain. However, there is very little agreement among the various dental specialities about the nature, causes and treatment, so that the majority of practicing dentists are in a dilemma about how to treat a patient who presents to them with a variety of complaints that can be attributed to TMJ dysfunction.

At the base of this dilemma is the concept that all "TMJ patients" are suffering the effects of a clinical entity which is described as a syndrome. There basically exists two such syndrome theories and the treatment a patient receives will depend upon which theory the practicing dentist follows.

## The myofascial pain dysfunction syndrome (MPD)

The exponents of the myofascial pain dysfunction syndrome have concluded that the etiology is emotional stress. This syndrome is defined as consisting of 4 cardinal symptoms: pain, muscular tenderness, limitation of jaw movement and clicking. Exponents of the MPD syndrome have observed that most patients with these symptoms have increased emotional stress as revealed by psychological testing and elevated levels of 17-hydroxysteroids and catecholamines. These are not sufficient objective criteria to blame emotional stress for a set of symptoms which include objective signs. MPD articles have dealt almost entirely with the subjective symptoms and have failed to provide a satisfactory explanation for the objective signs. These objective signs are limitation of jaw opening and clicking. They can be measured and recorded by several clinical methods. These objective signs of the MPD syndrome are also signs of a displaced articular disc.

## The TMJ occlusal dysfunction syndrome

During the past 3 decades, there has been an increasing interest in the concept that irregular dental occlusion is the primary cause of TMJ symptoms. However, among the exponents of this syndrome there is no real agreement about the relationship of the position of the dental occlusion to the condylar position. As dentists we tend to be precise and use instruments which are extremely precise in measuring and recording mandibular movements and condylar positions. Considering this and the fact that there are many differing views about the ideal relationship between intercuspal position and the position of the condyles in the fossa, we must question the significance of a precise relationship between centric occlusion (CO) and centric relation (CR). The universal biological observation that nature is not precise in morphology and function can apply to the relationship between CO and CR. Many TMJ patients are benefitted by occlusal treatment but a significant number are not, and some get much worse.

So there exists a dilemma in the management of TMJ patients. The profession is largely divided into 2 camps and the proponents of MPD syndrome cannot adequately explain the objective symptoms and the occlusionists cannot explain their failures.

The signs and symptoms vary greatly among TMJ patients. Some have clicking joints while others have a grinding noise. Some patients have tenderness in the joints, others in the muscles and some have tenderness in both. Most have headaches and some will complain of ear noise. Many have a combination of pain in the joints and limited movement, while others have limited movement without pain. Still others have no limitation of movement, no clicking but severe headaches. Now, a syndrome is a concurrence of signs and symptoms, and *since TMJ patients present such a variety of signs and symptoms, to say a patient has a TMJ syndrome is not accurate.* The idea that TMJ patients are suffering from a common syndrome has resulted in attempts to determine what they have in common rather than how and why they are different. The idea of an all-inclusive syndrome must be discarded. Most TMJ articles appearing in the dental literature assign TMJ patients to a single category without regard to differentiation. At the base of any good diagnosis, no matter what the condition, is the differential diagnosis. The same holds true for TMJ patients. There are many different categories into which TMJ patients may be placed. The point here is that to only consider one or two "syndromes", lumping all patients into them and treating accordingly is poor practice.

### Differential Diagnosis

TMJ problems can be broadly classified as developmental abnormalities, diseases, and dysfunctions.

*The developmental abnormalities* include hypoplasia, hyperplasia, impingement of the coronoid process, chondromas, and ossification of ligaments such as Eagles syndrome.

*The intracapsular diseases* include degenerative arthritis, osteochondritis, rheumatoid arthritis, psoriatic arthritis, synovial chondromotosis, infections, steroid necrosis, gout and metastatic tumors. Differentiation must also be made within this category. Most of these conditions have phases or stages in which the clinical symptoms vary greatly. For example, rheumatoid arthritis has 4 stages and there are 3 basic types of degenerative arthritis. Diagnosis must include clinical knowledge of the various developmental abnormalities and diseases and the characteristics of their various stages.

*Dysfunctions* are abnormal conditions that are neither developmental abnormalities nor diseases. They may be manifestations of these but can also occur as separate entities.

### Intracapsular Dysfunctions

There are several intracapsular dysfunctions which may afflict the TMJ. One is intracapsular edema or posterior capsulitis. Here the highly vascular posterior capsular ligament becomes inflamed and edema builds up in the joint space. Typically, the mandible will deviate toward the affected side in maximal opening and toward the opposite side during rest. Retruding the mandible causes a significant amount of pain. The edema may be caused by infection, arthritic inflammation and trauma of extrinsic and intrinsic origin. Often this is the first stage of another intracapsular dysfunction – displacement of the articular disc (internal derangement) of the TMJ. The remainder of this paper will be devoted to this one dysfunction, which, by our account, is responsible for 80% of all TMJ problems. We will discuss under the following sections:

(A) Nature of disc displacement
(B) Causes
(C) History and clinical examination
(D) Diagnosis
(E) Treatment

## (A) Nature of displacement of the articular disc (Internal Derangement)

Neither the proponents of the MPD syndrome nor the occlusal dysfunction syndrome take into account the position and the condition of the articular disc in explaining their theories. Yet the disc is in the center of the joint, interposed between the temporal bone and condyle. That the disc serves a definite function has been largely overlooked in both the literature and in practice. Dysfunction and displacement of the disc, however, have been well described in the literature, particularly the British.[1, 2, 3] More recently the dysfunction has been described by many others.[4–10] I will attempt to amplify on what has previously been written about disc displacement and describe the diagnostic methodology of the displaced disc as we see it in Montgomery, Alabama in treating patients.

In order to understand an abnormal TMJ one must know and understand the function of a normal joint. Useful information can be gained from the transcranial radiograph. In examining the normal transcranial radiograph (Fig. 1) we basically see three components, these being the condyle, the temporal bone (fossa) and the space between these two. Too often this space has been neglected for failure to realize that the seemingly empty space on the radiograph actually contains the radiolucent articular disc and its ligamentous attachments. Although the disc cannot be seen on the radiograph, its position can be inferred by the relative position of the condyle to the fossa. Note on the normal radiograph that the condyle in the closed jaw position is seated concentrically within the fossa and there is at least 2mm of joint space. Here the disc and attachments are in a normal position. In this X-ray the bony architecture of both the temporal bone and condyle are normal. The central position of the fossa is concave with a good layer of cortical bone and the condyle shows an absence of spurring, anterior beaking, or flattening, and likewise shows a good cortical bone layer.

Internal derangement (displacement of the disc) is defined as an anterior displacement of the disc associated with posterior–sup-

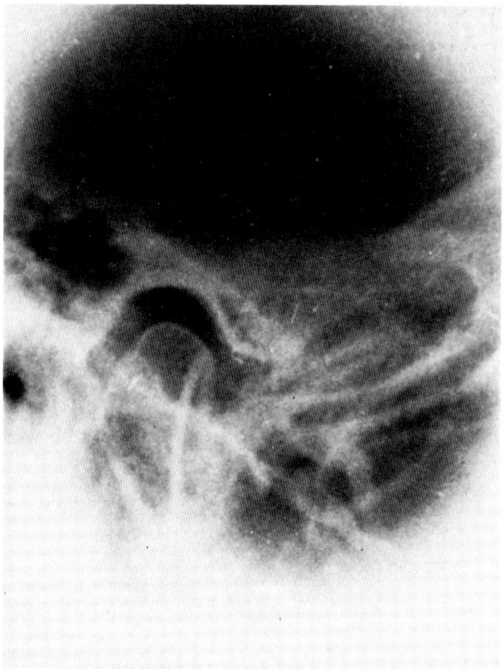

Fig. 1 Normal transcranial radiograph. The condyle has a concentric relationship with respect to the mandibular fossa which is radiographic evidence that the articular disc is in its correct relationship to the mandibular condyle, in the closed jaw position.

erior displacement of the condyle in the closed jaw position. Diagnosing from radiographic evidence alone, if the relative position of the condyle to the fossa changes in the closed jaw position, then the position of the disc **must** be changed also.

Figure 2A schematically shows the three elements of the joint, the condyle, the fossa, disc and attachment. Note the concentricity of the condyle to the fossa with the disc interposed. Posteriorly the disc is held in place by the posterior attachment or ligament. This ligament is composed of both elastic and non-elastic tissue, blends anteriorly into the disc proper and posteriorly attaches to the condyle inferiorly and the temporal bone superiorly. The posterior edge of the disc is located just at the superior–posterior aspect of the condyle. The posterior attachment is very vascular and is prone to being overstretched.

If the joint is subjected to trauma and the vector of force is such that the condyle is driven postero-superiorly, the posterior attachment will stretch and the articular disc will migrate anteriorly (Fig. 2B). Radiographically you will see a decrease in the posterior joint space. If this trauma continues, the attachment will become more stretched, thinner and weaker, and the disc will migrate even farther anteriorly (Fig. 2C). Radiographically the postero-superior displacement of the condyle is seen in Figure 3.

With such a narrow posterior joint space, the disc **must** be located anterior to the condyle. The disc is loose, out of normal position and will click and pop on jaw movement. The direction and magnitude of displacement can be measured by several different methods which will be discussed later.

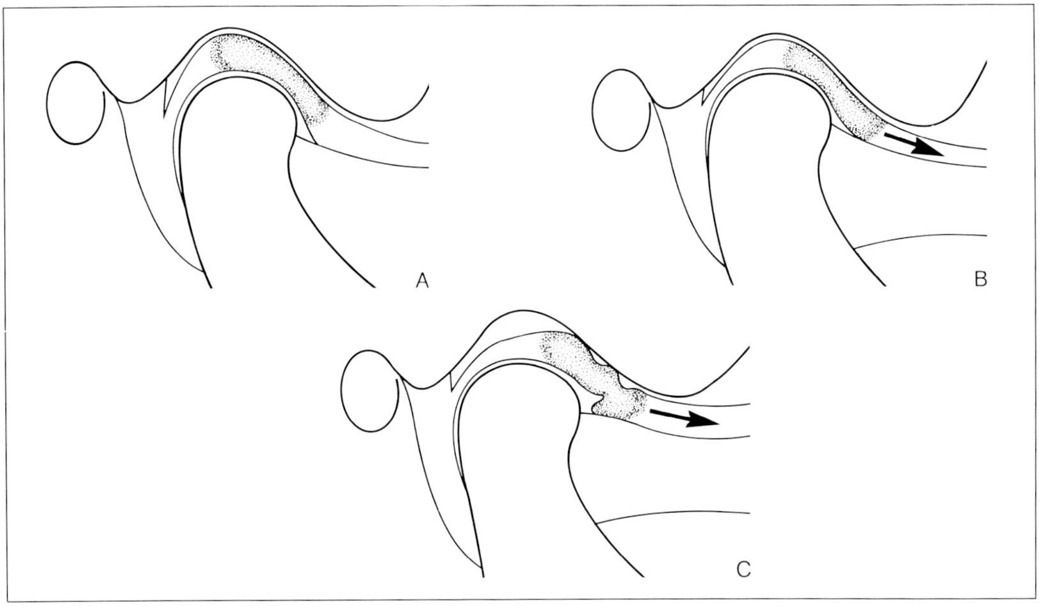


Fig. 2
A. Normal relationship of the condyle to the articular disc, and temporal bone.
B. Articular disc is slightly displaced.
C. Advanced displacement of the articular disc.

**The closed lock**

When the thick posterior portion of the disc becomes displaced completely anteriorly to the condyle, it will serve as a mechanical block or impingement to jaw opening. The disc will be jammed between the condyle and the articular eminence, prohibiting normal condylar translation. This is referred to as the closed-lock. In the closed-lock the patient will typically open to around 25 mm and the joint **will not click** (Fig. 4, 5). Although some secondary muscle spasm may exist, the closed-lock should not be mistaken for muscular trismus and can be confirmed by history and radiographs. If left untreated or improperly treated, the posterior attachment will stretch even farther and the probability of a tear or perforation in the attachment is increased.

Internal derangement must be looked upon as a continuing process. In treating patients, the clinician will obviously see the process at only one stage in its spectrum from initial injury to complete breakdown of the joint. Typically, the initial insult to the joint displaces the condyle posteriorly, with concomitant stretching of the posterior attachment and anterior displacement of the disc. The joint will usually be sore and have some degree of intracapsular edema. Clicking will begin as the disc is now loose and it will be of an intermittent or continuing nature. The clicks will occur at different points of jaw opening, depending upon how far anteriorly the disc is displaced. If the click occurs early in jaw opening the degree of anterior displacement is small, whereas a click occuring close to the maximal opening position would indicate the disc has been displaced farther anteriorly. When the degree in displacement becomes

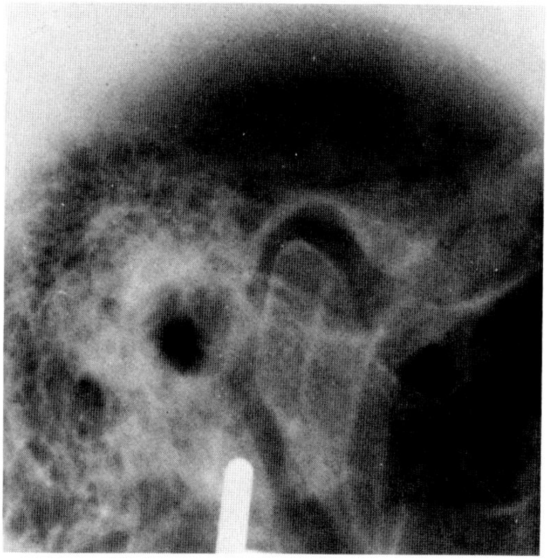

Fig. 3 Transcranial oblique radiograph showing posterior displacement of the condyle, indicating that the articular disc has been displaced anteriorly while the posterior attachment has been stretched and thinned.

such that the disc lodges anterior to the condyle, the patient will experience locking. This may be intermittent with the patient experiencing clicking and locking, or the patient may go into a permanent closed-lock. Under a permanent closed-lock condition, jaw opening will increase but the disc will still be lodged anteriorly to the condyle and jaw opening is increased at the expense of stretching the posterior attachment, which is subject to tearing. *One must therefore distinguish between an acute and chronic closed-lock as, clinically, they are quite different.* When the disc is displaced, the bony elements of the joint are not protected by the cushioning effect of the disc and degenerative changes begin. Left untreated or improperly treated the end result is degenerative arthritis and the probability that the posterior attachment of the disc will become perforated.

## (B) Causes

There are many causes for disc displacement and they can, in general, be placed into two broad categories, being acute or chronic trauma.

**Acute:** This category would include sudden traumatic episodes which displace the condyle posteriorly or stretch the posterior attachment and in effect loosen the disc. An example would be trauma to the mandible as a result of an accident or excessive force applied to the jaw during extraction of teeth or intubation. This is especially true if the joint is already compromised.

**Chronic:** This category would include low grade microtrauma over a long period of time. Examples here would include any forces which cause the mandible to move into a retruded position. Here we would consider loss of posterior teeth, incisal interference, occlusal contacts which deflect the jaw posteriorly and iatrogenic causes.
To give one example, let us consider the retentive phase of typical orthodontic therapy. In a premolar extraction case, when the orthodontic bands are removed, a labial retention wire is placed on the upper arch

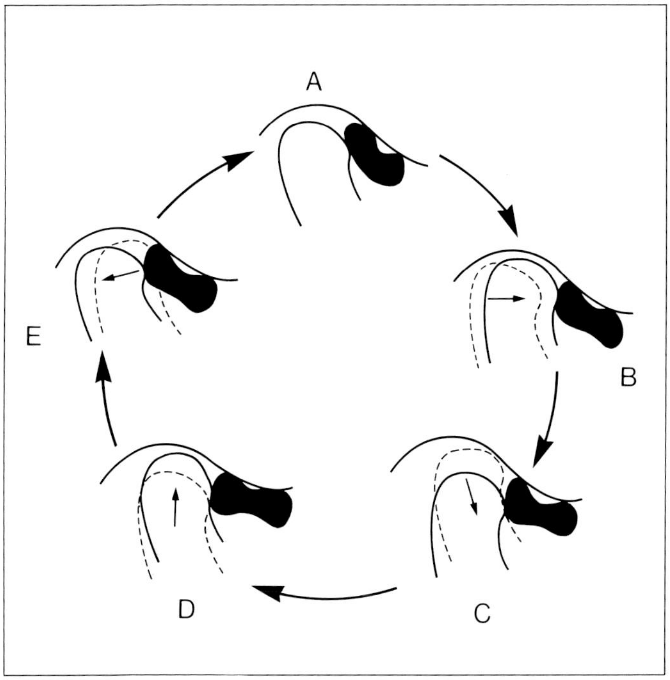


Fig. 4 Diagram showing the disc relationship in the clinical closed lock. The articular disc remains displaced anteriorly with respect to the condyle in all movements. The condyle is observed to be distracted from the temporal bone on maximal opening.

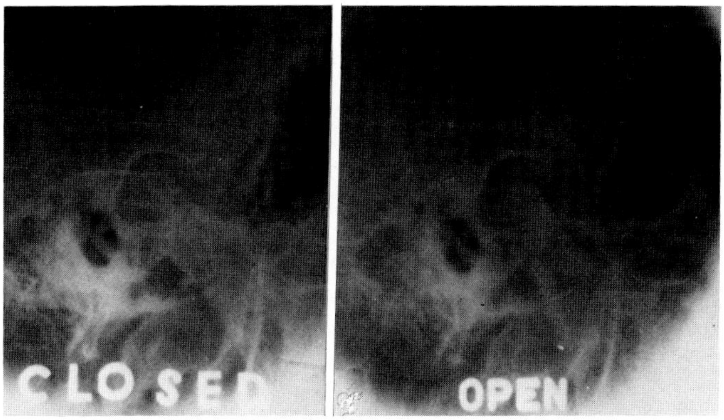


Fig. 5 A. In the transcranial radiograph in the closed lock position, the condyle appears to be in a retruded relationship. The joint space is reduced posteriorly and superiorly. This is suggestive of anterior displacement of the disc. B. Wide open position (24 mm). Here, the movement of the condyle is limited because of the jamming effect of the thickened disc. Notice that the vertical joint space is *increased*.

and a lingual wire is placed on the lower arch. The posterior teeth then settle, decreasing the vertical dimension of occlusion, and the lower anterior teeth are driven onto the lingual surfaces of the upper anteriors. The vector of force is now generated to drive the condyles posteriorly and the process previously described begins (Fig. 6). Similarly if during extensive reconstruction the occlusion is set with the condyles functioning at the posterior border positions the disc may become displaced. This may happen if the bite registration is made with the mandible in a retruded position (centric relation). This is particularly likely to occur if the patient is in a reclining position where gravity alone will

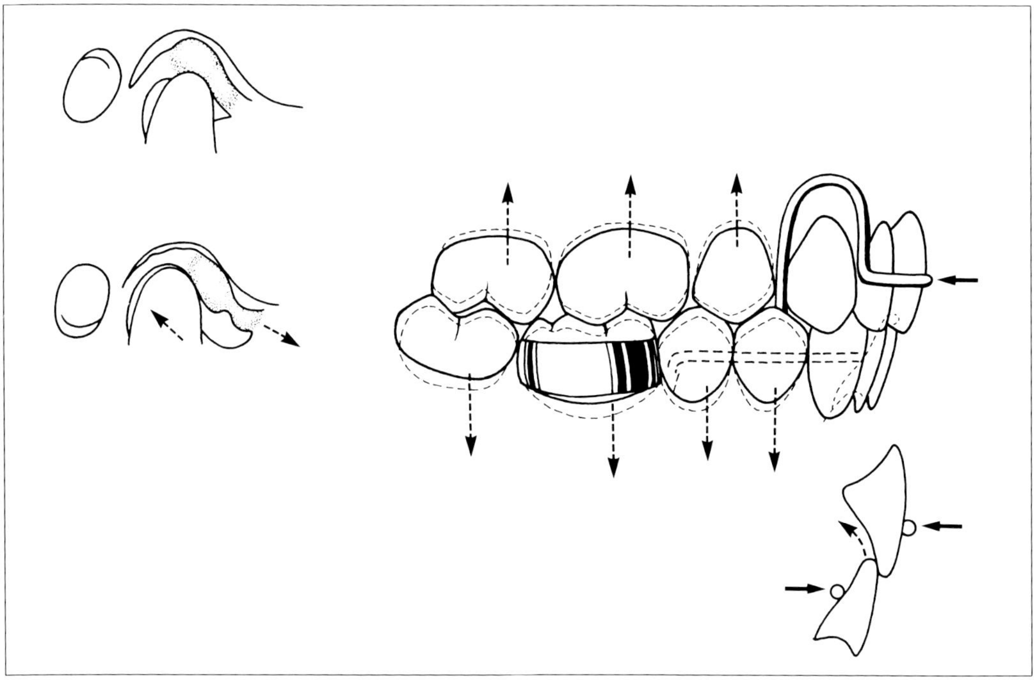

Fig. 6 Etiology of anterior displacement of the articular disc from chronic trauma. For example, this could occur if posterior support were lost during the retention phase of orthodontic treatment. This would result in a relative and opposite displacement of the condyle and articular disc.

retrude the mandible. Most disc displacements are not related to dental treatment; however, if the condyles are retruded on a patient with a displaced disc, the dysfunction is aggravated.

## (C) History and clinical exam

Listening to the history of a TMJ patient is quite laborious. However, it has often been said that if a clinician listens well enough and is armed with enough knowledge, the patient will tell you what is wrong. More often than not, amid usually lengthy histories, similar patterns and complaints will emerge. Most of the following signs and symptoms typify the examination of TMJ patients.

### Pain

Pain is variable in intensity, duration and location. The most striking location is retro-orbital. It also occurs in the temporal, occipital and shoulder areas. There may be pain directly over the joint but this is not as frequent as the retro-orbital location. Pain may be intermittent with advanced cases being more continuous.

### Earache

In reality the earache is pain in the joint due to the juxtaposition of the TMJ and ear canal. The canal should be inspected with an otoscope and if a problem is apparent, consultation with an ear specialist should be obtained.

### Headache

Because headache, retro-orbital, temporal and occipital pain are the most common complaints among TMJ patients, a close working relationship with a neurologist is necessary. The neurologists see many headache patients in which a dysfunctional TMJ is responsible for their presenting symptoms. On the other hand any patient whose presenting symptoms are headache related should have a neurological consultation. Some patients actually have 2 types of headaches concomitantly, one from the TMJ and one neurological. Also to be considered, in cases of temporal headaches is a relatively elongated coronoid process which is often symptomatic particularly in cases of disc displacement. Injections of an anesthetic solution at the tip of the coronoid process will confirm this.

### Limited Opening

The closed-lock typically limits the mandibular opening to around 25—30 mm in the acute cases. Increased opening will develop with chronicity. The limitation is most often misdiagnosed as trismus. Most patients will relate past clicking and sudden limitation of opening. Trismus can be ruled out by manipulating the mandible, a maneuver which will be described later. In addition, etiological factors for trismus such as infected teeth must be ruled out. Occasionally a patient with a closed-lock may have some degree of muscle spasm but usually this is secondary to the mechanical jamming effect of the displaced disc.

### Limited Lateral Movement

When the disc becomes dislocated anteriorly and jams the joint, lateral excursion to the opposite side is limited. If the right disc is dislocated, lateral movement will be limited to the left side.

### Deviation

Similarly, when the disc is dislocated the mandible will deviate toward the affected side in the position of maximal opening. If the right disc is dislocated the mandible will deviate to the right on opening.

### Noise

Noise is a sign of an unhealthy joint. By listening to the joint, the clinician can gain insight to the patho-physiology and degree of dysfunction and disease. Joint noise can be heard with the ear alone or with a stethoscope, and felt by a palpating finger placed over the joint. The most common type of joint noise will be described as reciprocal clicking or popping. The opening click occurs when the condyle, moving beneath the disc and posterior attachment, snaps under the posterior band of the disc and seats in its normal position beneath the disc. The closing click occurs near the terminus of the closing movement and is made as the condyle slips posterior to the posterior band of the disc, and the disc becomes displaced anteriorly. *In a nutshell, the closing click results in disc displacement and the opening click occurs as he disc is snapped back into normal position.* This is known as *reciprocal clicking* and will be discussed later.

A *grinding noise* is indicative of degenerative arthritis and is heard mostly on translation and seldom on rotation. *A grating or cracking noise* indicates advanced degenerative arthritis and must be distinguished from clicking and popping. Experience in listening to joints plus other diagnostic methods will help differentiate between a moderately displaced disc and advanced degenerative arthritis with a possible perforation of the posterior attachment. There is one important thing to remember about joint noise. *The joint that clicks is not locked and the joint that is locked does not click.* So, the dysfunctional joint will make certain sounds from clicking to grinding to cracking which will indicate the stage of the dysfunction. Reciprocal clicking can be graded and this indicates the degree of displacement of the disc, which is valuable to the diagnosis and ultimate treatment plan. The grading of reciprocal clicks will be discussed under the section on diagnosis.

There are other signs and symptoms which many TMJ patients will relate such as numbness in the arm on the effected side and noise in the ear. Patients will often say "There is water dripping in my ear" or "It sounds like there is a cricket in my ear". Some patients will have atypical neuralgias which are relieved when the disc is relocated into its proper position.

## (D) Diagnosis

The best diagnostic tools are the history and examination. This must be supplemented by a good working differential diagnosis and by other specific studies. The clinician should look for causative factors in the history, the signs and symptoms previously discussed, and formulate an idea as to the stage of the dysfunction based on knowledge of the pathophysiology. There are several other tools available to the clinician to make the diagnosis of a displaced disc and correlate the results to the presenting symtoms.

### Radiographs

Radiographic studies will include transcranial oblique films, both lateral and antero-posterior head films, orthopantomograms, tomograms and arthrograms.

A good lateral, transcranial film of the TM joints is the number one diagnostic tool in addition to the history and examination. No patient should ever be treated for a TMJ problem without transcranial films. To do so is as good a practice as filling or extracting teeth without a dental radiograph. The films should be of good quality and show the closed, rest and open positions. They should be taken by the clinician and one should not depend on the hospital for several reasons. Hospital films of the TMJ are generally of poor quality in angulation. The closed position must be taken with the teeth completely together (position of maximal intercuspation); X-ray technicians may fail to do this. Radiologists are usually looking for gross pathology, such as severe degenerative arthritis, advanced rheumatoid arthritis and fractures. Usually they will not look closely at the spatial relationship of the condyle to the fossa, and a narrowed posterior joint space may be read out as normal.

In the transcranial films we are looking for deviation from the concentrically seated condyle in the closed position with an adequate joint space of at least 2 mm. A retruded condyle with a narrow postero-superior joint space is diagnostic. Often one will see a shortened condyle on one side because of degenerative arthritis and a painfully displaced disc on the opposite. This frequently occurs because the asymptomatic arthritic side has shortened causing the ligaments to stretch on the opposite side, displacing the disc.

Degenerative arthritis is the end point of a displaced disc and here one will see a reduced joint space, flattening or irregular articulating surfaces of the condyle and fossa and sclerosis of the condyle, mandibular neck and fossa.

Antero-posterior films facilitate the observation of irregularities of the lateral and medial poles and superior surface of the condyle. Orthopantomograms are of little value other than for observing the shortening or hy-

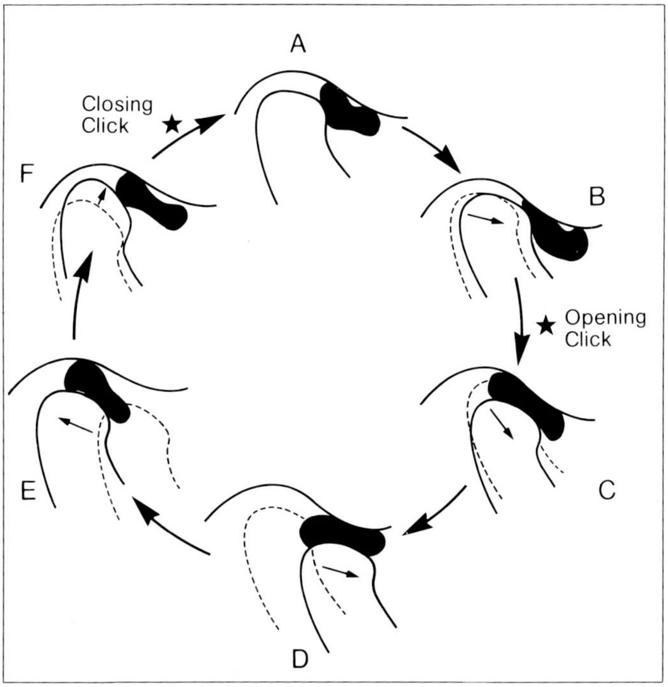


Fig. 7 Schematic of reciprocal clicking. Asterisk represents the point where the clicking sound occurs on opening and closing.

perplasia of the condyle, the size and shape of the coronoid processes and other conditions such as antigonial notching etc.

Tomographic studies are excellent, but probably impractical for all patients. A diagnosis of a displaced disc can be made without tomography if the transcranial films are of good quality and the other diagnostic studies are performed correctly. Although the transcranial film reveals only the lateral one half of the joint, I believe it is the best single radiographic projection.

Arthrograms provide specific criteria to determine the normal and abnormal positions of the disc in its relationship to the condyle in varying degrees of condylar translation. Arthrograms can be correlated with condylographic studies in determining the degree of displacement of the disc. Prior to discussing these two diagnostic studies one must have a firm conception of reciprocal clicking and locking. This has been discussed but will be repeated because of its importance.

In reciprocal clicking the opening click occurs at a point located somewhere in the protrusive path. When the click occurs during opening, the condyle suddenly snaps forward and the disc snaps backward into its normal position. The closing click occurs near the end of the retrusive condyle movement. When the click occurs during closing, the condyle snaps suddenly upward and backward and the disc becomes displaced anteriorly. **Reciprocal clicking** is classified as **early, intermediate** or **late,** depending upon the degree of opening at which the click occurs. In reciprocal clicking the closing click will not occur unless it is preceeded by the opening click. Figure 7 is a schematic of reciprocal clicking. At the 12 o'clock position the teeth are occluded and the disc is dis-

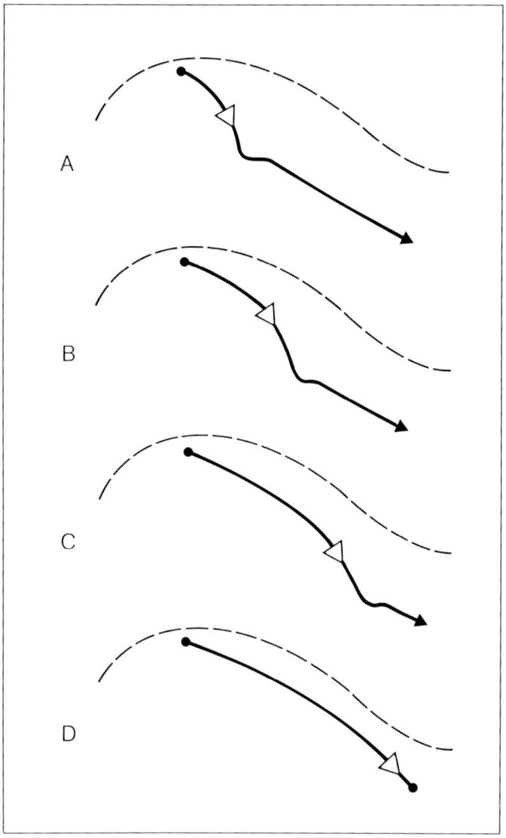


Fig. 8 Condylar path measurements transposed to line drawings (after *Farrar*).

A. early. B. intermediate, and C. late clicks. D. tracing of a patient with chronic lock, which is very similar to a normal tracing.

placed anteriorly. Remember the definition of internal derangement. As the condyle translates forward the disc is still anteriorly displaced until the 4 o'clock position where the click occurs and the disc snaps into place. It is in place until the closing click occurs between 8 and 10 o'clock and the disc is again displaced anteriorly. As reciprocal clicking becomes more chronic, the opening click begins to occur at a point closer to the open position. Eventually the disc remains continuously anteriorly dislocated throughout the full range of condylar translation.

In locking, the disc remains dislocated anteriorly and jams the condyle, causing limitation of opening in the acute stage. As locking becomes more chronic, the range of movement gradually increases because the condyle begins to push the dislocated disc farther, at the risk of tearing the posterior attachment.

Figure 8 shows condylar path measurements transposed to line drawings, showing early, intermediate and late clicks (Fig. 8A, B, C). Figure 8D shows a chronic closed-lock which is very similar to a normal tracing. Here the history, radiographs and arthrograms confirm the diagnosis.

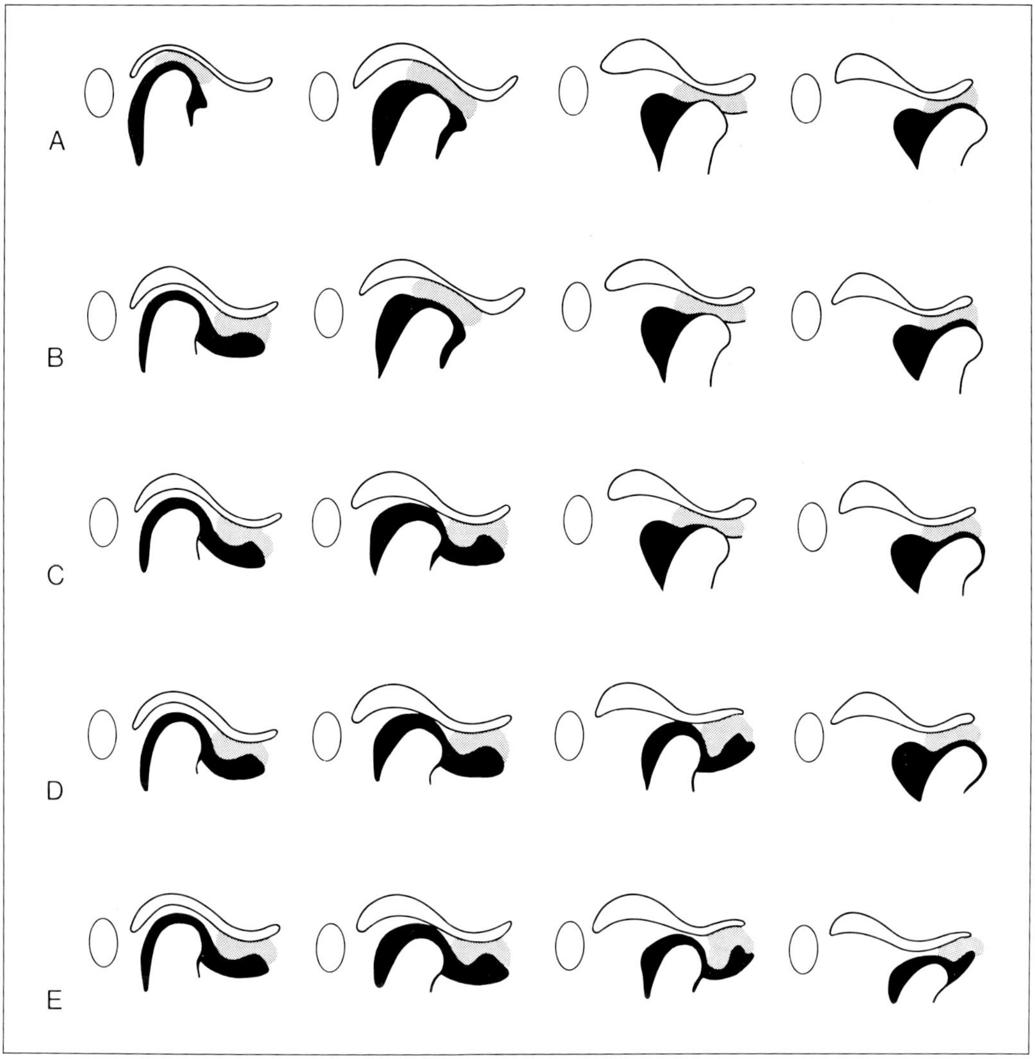


Fig. 9 Line drawings taken from numerous arthrograms showing articular disc displacement at various points of condyle movement.

A. normal joint. B. early opening click. C. intermediate opening click. D. late opening click. E. complete anterior dislocation of the articular disc or closed lock.

## Arthrograms

If a small amount of water soluble contrast medium is injected into both the upper and lower joint spaces, the articular disc and attachment will be outlined and its position can be noted throughout the complete range of mandibular movement. However, only the inferior space needs to be cannulated and filled to determine the normal and abnormal positions of the disc in its relationship to the condyle during translation.

In a normal joint in the closed position, the posterior portion of the inferior joint space is concave-convex. The convex posterior outline corresponds to the inner surface of the posterior attachment which is attached to the condyle. The concave aspect outlines the posterior surface of the condyle. Anteriorly, a small amount of contrast medium is extruded into the lower anterior recess. When the condyle moves forward the posterior portion gradually changes form and developes a sigmoid shape caused by bulging of the posterior attachment just behind the thick posterior band of the disc. At the same time, the small amount of contrast medium anteriorly begins to be evacuated into the posterior space. As the condyle moves forward to maximum opening, the sigmoid shape becomes more pronounced and almost all of the contrast medium is evacuated from the anterior to the posterior space. When the disc is displaced anteriorly the contrast medium remains in the anterior compartment and the posterior space does not assume the characteristic sigmoid shape.

Figure 9 shows the line drawings taken from numerous arthrograms showing displacement occuring at various points in translation. Figure 9A shows a normal joint. The black area of the inferior space will be seen as white on the actual arthrogram, since it is filled with contrast medium. The stippled area is the position of the disc. Notice the small amount of contrast in the anterior compartment and the characteristic sigmoid shaped formed posteriorly as the condyle translates forward. Figure 9 B shows an early click. Reading from left to right the disc is displaced anteriorly. A large amount of contrast medium is in the anterior compartment. As the condyle moves forward the click occurs, contrast medium is evacuated from anterior to posterior, the sigmoid shape forms and the disc is in its normal position for the remainder of the opening. Figures 9C and 9D show intermediate and late opening clicks. Figure 9E shows a complete anterior dislocation or closed-lock. If acute, the opening will be limited and will gradually increase over a period of time.

Arthrograms can be correlated with condylar path measurements as shown in Figure 10. Figure 10A shows a line drawing of a normal arthrogram and the corresponding normal condylar path tracing. Figure 10B illustrates an intermediate click and Figures 10C and 10D show complete anterior dislocation of the articular discs. The condylar path tracing in Figure 10C is characteristic of an acute closed-lock with limited opening, while Figure 10D is characteristic of a chronic closed-lock or complete anterior dislocation showing a normal, or perhaps excessive, opening range. Note that this condylar path tracing is similar to the normal pathway. Again, I must emphasize, transcranial films, history and arthrograms will make the diagnosis.

**Manipulation**

This is another diagnostic technique which will also serve as a treatment modality. Typically a patient with locking will present, to the office saying, "My jaw used to click and pop, but now it won't open all the way". If locking has occured within 3 or 4 weeks the jaw can usually be manipulated by distracting the condyle and pulling it forward and medially (Fig. 11). When successful, the joint will snap when the disc returns to its normal position and full range of movement is instantaneously restored. An occlusal splint which repositions the mandible anteriorly should be placed immediately. Even with the appliance the disc may become completely dislocated again. Even if the disc does not stay in position for any length of time, this maneuver will prove the dislocated disc is the cause of

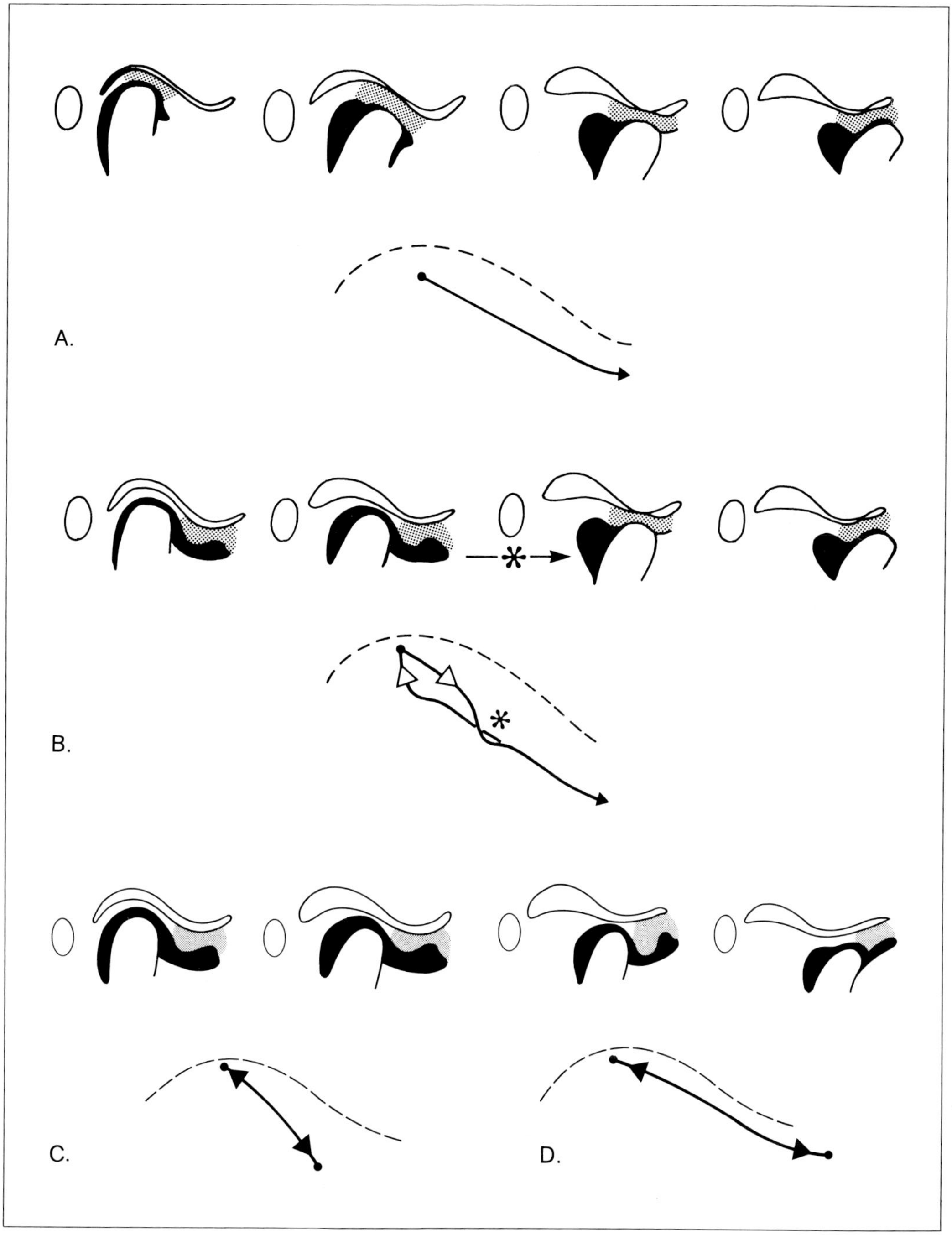


Fig. 10 Arthrogram correlated with condyle path measurement.
A. Normal condyle. B. Intermediate click. C. Complete anterior dislocation of the articular disc.

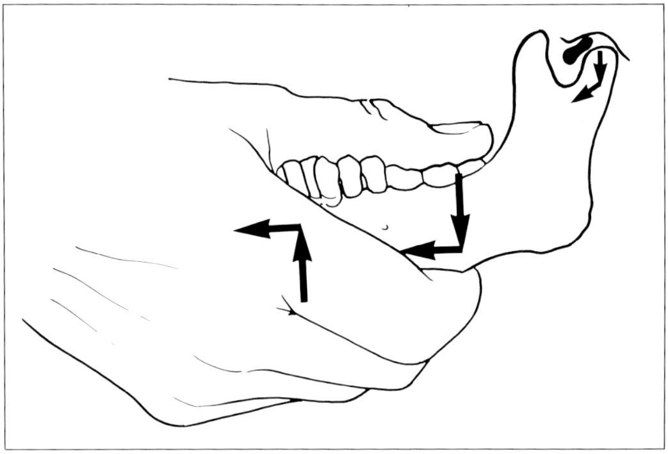

Fig. 11 Manipulation of the locked jaw by distracting the condyle and pulling it forward and medially.

limited movement and thus, will rule out trismus.

To summarize, the diagnosis of a TMJ patient should include a history, examination and good quality transcranial oblique films. The diagnosis of anterior displacement of the disc can be confirmed and detailed with condylar path measurements, arthrograms and manipulation.

## (E) Treatment

Once the diagnosis of anterior disc displacement has been established a treatment plan must be instituted. In general, the extensiveness of treatment will depend upon the severity of the symptoms, and upon the success of conservative therapy. Treatment is directed at restoring the displaced disc back to its normal position, and ranges from equilibration of the teeth, bite plane therapy, cast dental restorations, and orthodontics to surgery.

Treatment should be undertaken using a team approach, consisting of a team leader, normally a general dentist well versed in occlusion and TMJ dysfunction, an orthodontist and an oral surgeon. The team should have a good working relationship with a neurologist or neurosurgeon.

Eighty percent of the patients with anterior disc displacement can be managed successfully with consevative treatment. The chronicity of the dysfunction and the amount of displacement as well as the stability of the occlusion are indices of the predicted success of conservative treatment. An early click is easily treated by changing the occlusal position whereas a late click, complete dislocation, advanced degenerative arthritis of the progressive type and perforated or torn posterior attachments are surgical cases if the symptoms are severe.

Since the condyle has been displaced postero-superiorly, conservative treatment is directed toward positioning the condyle anteriorly in the fossa, allowing the disc to slip posteriorly into its normal position. In other words, attempt to reverse the process of dysfunction. This may be accomplished by removal of tooth contacts which deflect the mandible posteriorly, or the forward repositioning of the affected condyle with crowns or onlays or orthodontics. Incisal interference may be eliminated with orthodontic therapy and surgery. The main-

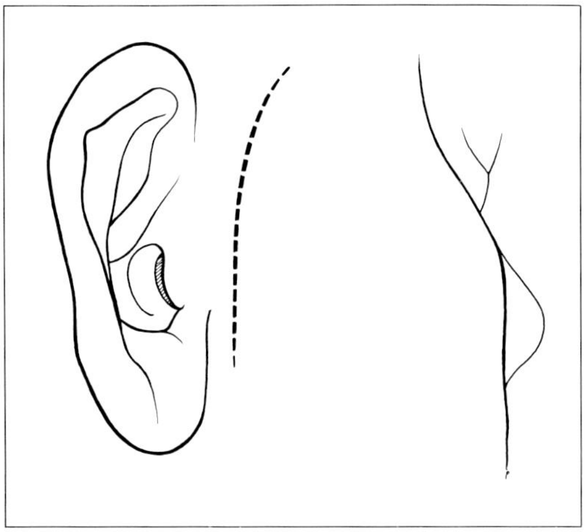

Fig. 12 A preauricular incision is made with a slight curve; the dissection is carried down to the temporalis fascia and around the external auditory canal. The parotid gland is retracted out of the way.

stay of corrective treatment is the full coverage maxillary jaw repositioning appliance. This appliance will reposition the retruded condyle or condyles forward and "capture" the displaced disc. Following the initial phase with the jaw repositioning appliance, more permanent reconstruction is undertaken if the disc has remained in place for 2–3 months. In addition, missing posterior teeth must be replaced. If more conservative treatment does not yield favorable results and surgery is anticipated, all occlusal factors which will cause the condyle to be retruded must be eliminated.

## Surgery

When conservative treatment fails, surgery is considered if the symptoms are of such a quality, intensity and constancy to warrant an invasive procedure. Surgery alone is seldom sufficient and the surgeon must work closely with the occlusionist when investigating the etiology of the dysfunction. Once the dysfunction has advanced to a certain point, only repair of the joint may reverse the process which, in the majority of cases, began with an occlusion which retruded the condyle. Therefore, if surgery is successful and the faulty occlusion is not corrected, the case will ultimately fail. Reconstructive arthroplasty is directed at repair of the damaged joint, using what is there and avoiding placement of synthetic materials such as silastic and metallic devices.

The stretched and thinned posterior attachment is transected, the postero-superior aspect of the condyle is reduced and smoothed and the disc is reconstructed to the posterior attachment in its normal position. Figures 12 to 17 are illustrations of a typical surgical case. Success or failure of surgery is based on both subjective and objective criteria. Paramount is the elimination of pain. Probably any surgical procedure which invades the joint will provide temporary relief as the joint has been partially denervated. However, both the patient and surgeon are looking for lasting results. If the reconstructive arthroplasty is performed correctly and the occlusion is stable, to prevent retrusion of the condyle, long lasting relief of both the signs and symptoms of internal derangement can be expected.

Objectively, success can be measured by range of movement, deviation and joint

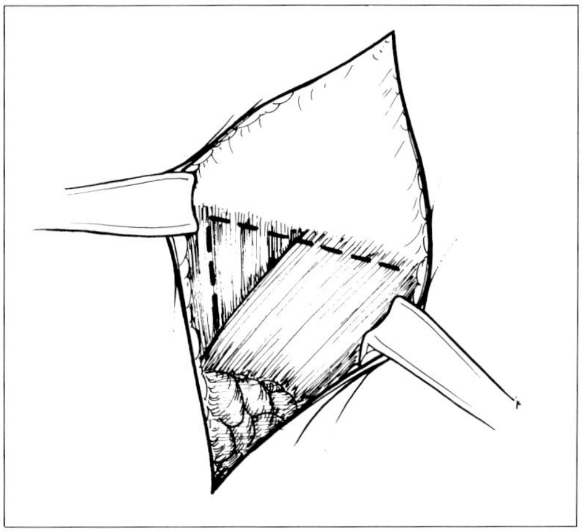

Fig. 13 An incision is made below the zygomatic arch horizontally and slightly vertically posteriorly *through the capsule*. Branches of the facial nerve are contained in the anterior flap.

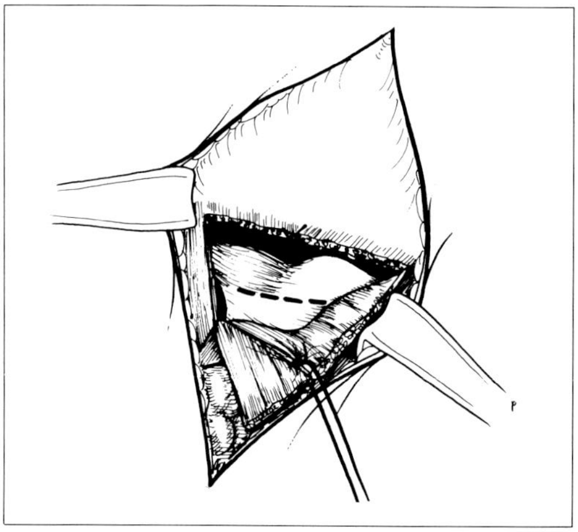

Fig. 14 The capsule is "taken down" in an anterior-inferior direction, exposing the upper joint space, superior surfaces and lateral wall of disc. An incision is made through the lateral wall of the disc to enter the lower joint space.

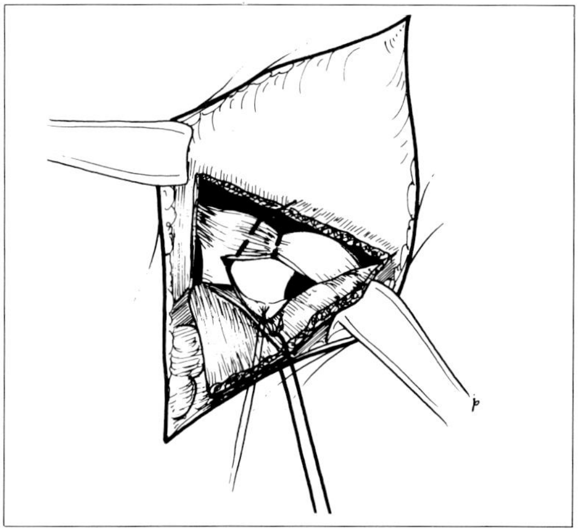

Fig. 15 Dissection defines the disc and stretched posterior attachment and exposes the condyle.

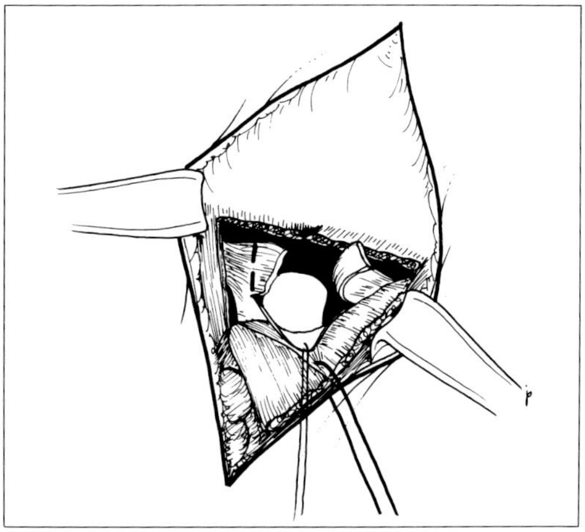

Fig. 16 The posterior attachment is transected from lateral to medial near its junction to the disc proper and the condyle is adequately exposed for reduction and smoothening of the posterior aspect. A portion of the stretched posterior attachment is removed.

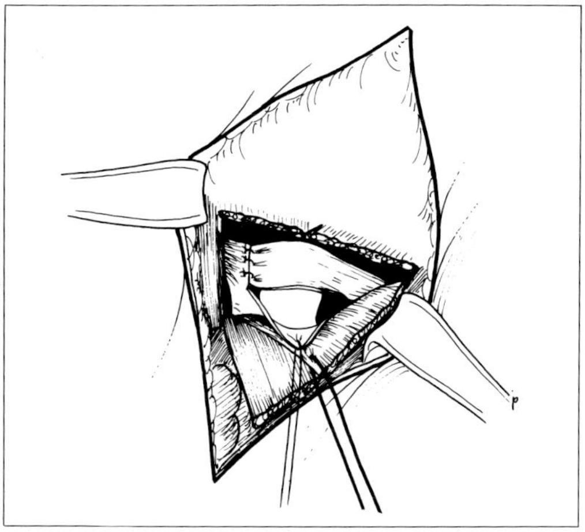

Fig. 17 The disc is sutured to the posterior attachment and tested for strength of the suture line. The lateral wall of the disc and capsule are then sutured and the incision is closed.

noise; subjectively, by relief of temporal, occipital and retro-orbital pain. In cases of tears of the disc-posterior attachment and even complete perforations, the joint is repaired. The disc should not be removed.

## Summary

TMJ problems are complex and often difficult to diagnose and treat. They cannot be simplified into one or two syndrome theories but encompass a variety of developmental abnormalities, diseases and dysfunctions. The majority of TMJ patients are suffering from the dysfunction of a displacement of the articular disc. These patients have common signs and symptoms including clicking, locking, retro-orbital, temporal and occipital pain. Displacement of the disc is diagnosed from history and clinical examination, transcranial radiographs, condylar path movement and arthrograms. Treatment is directed toward relocating and stabilizing the disc in its normal position by both occlusal and surgical methods. When members of both the dental and medical professions recognize the symptoms caused by internal derangement of the TMJ, we will find that this dysfunction is extremely prevalent. By a united effort among the various specialists and generalists we can improve upon the diagnosis and treatment and end or limit suffering in literally millions of people afflicted by temporomandibular pain and dysfunction.

### References


1. *Pringle, J. H.*
Displacement of the Mandibular Meniscus and its Treatment. Brit, J. of Surg. 6:385—389, 1918.

2. *Wakely, C.*
The Causation and Treatment of Displaced Mandibular Cartilage. Lancet 2:543—545, 1929.

3 *Ireland, V. E.*
"The Problem of the Clicking Jaw." Royal Soc. Med. 44:363—372, 1951 and Annals of Dent. 11:3—17, 1952.

4. *Kiehn, C. L.*
"Meniscectomy for Internal Derangement of Temporomandibular Joint." Amer. J. Surg. 364—373, 1952.

5. *Kiehn, C. L.* and *Des Prez, J. D.*
Meniscectomy for Internal Derangement of Temporomandibular Joint. Brit. J. Plast. Surg. 15:199—204, 1962.

6. *Silver, C. M.*, *Simon, S. D.* and *Savastano, A. A.*
"Meniscus Injuries of the Temporomandibular Joint." J. Bone Surg. 38—A:541—552, 1956.

7. *Silver, C. M.* and *Simon, S. D.*
"Meniscus Injuries of the Temporomandibular Joint: Further Experiences." J. Bone and Joint Surg. 45—A:113—124, 1963.

8. *Wilkes, C. H.*
"Structural and Functional Alterations of the Temporomandibular Joint," Northwest Dentistry, 57: 287-294, 1978.

9. *Farrar, W. B.*
"Diagnosis and Treatment of Painful Temporomandibular Joints." J. Prosthet. Dent. 20:345—351, 1968.

10. *Farrar, W. B.*
"Diagnosis and Treatment of Anterior Dislocation of the Articular Disc." N. Y. J. Dent. 40:348—351. 1971.


# Discussion

Discussant: Daniel Laskin

*Dr. Laskin*

I would like to take this opportunity to compliment Dr. *McCarty* on his presentation. I think he has brought our attention to a concept that perhaps has been overlooked. At least, I know I have overlooked this point. I have been aware for many years that people have talked about internal derangements. However, I have tended to put this concept aside, essentially because I have had difficulties dealing with it. Having made this statement, I would like to point out a few things with which I take issue. I think in any disease process there are two things we have to know: (1) we have to be able to diagnose the condition accurately, and (2) we have to understand the etiology. What we are doing here today, what we have been doing the last few years, and what we are looking forward to in the future is really refinement in these areas. We are just now beginning to understand what we are looking at in the arthrogram and, from the standpoint of diagnosis, we are just scratching the surface.

What conoerns me is that one can raise the same arguments against the concept of etiology of internal derangements as I have raised against dental occlusion being a primary factor in etiology of the MPD syndrome. What is causing all these internal derangements? I am not quite clear about it and it hasn't been explained to me. Why are most of the patients whom Dr. *McCarty* treats females? Why do females get more internal derangements than males? Why do you see this condition in a particular age group? These are questions which are unanswered. This is not being said in a critical way, but I feel we have to look at this whole process very thoughtfully. We have to be very careful in our selection of patients, and as we proceed we are going to learn. I would be very alarmed if I suddenly saw a trend toward surgical procedures for these problems. Does the oral surgeon who I used to think was very conservative, at least in recent years, suddenly become more aggressive because he has new operations? I would hate to see a spreading out of this concept so that everybody is trying it, rather than a few people with skill and expertise who have some background, like Dr. *McCarty* or Dr. *Wilkes,* or perhaps a few others in the country who would refine their concepts so that ultimately we can present the patient with a more logical approach to the problem than we can at the present time.

The other question that I would like to ask Dr. *McCarty* concerns whether he is treating clicking or pain? If he is treating clicking, I can understand one reason for his effectiveness because anytime you use an intracapsular operation you are tightening things up and you are going to reduce clicking. In terms of pain, I can only quote to you from *Toller's* article where he used an operation which was not quite the same but had similar connotations. He says that, "pain of intracapsular origin is very directly relieved by the nature of the incisions through the capsule, whereby the synovial membrane is deprived of afferent sensation and the nerve system mediating the reflex muscular control and tendency towards spasm, is directly interrupted to immediate clinical advantage." In many of our operations what we are doing when we relieve pain is denervating, and that is why historically you have seen many of these problems go away for a period of time and then come back as the nerve sensation returns.

The final comments I would like to make concern something which has been permeating the whole conference and that is the interpretation of the transcranial radiograph. Let me say that there is no way that people can make logical judgments about joint space from transcranial radiography. What you are looking at in a transcranial radiograph is the widest part of the condyle opposite the narrowest part of the fossa. If you think of the condyle as an irregular block of lead and you take a radiograph of an irregular object, you are going to get its widest image. If you think of the fossa as a megaphone made of lead, any way you shoot the X-ray beam through the megaphone, assuming that the film-target distance is not that large that you get wide divergence of the X-ray beam, will result in an image smaller than the large opening of the megaphone.

*Dr. Solberg*

In my opinion, one of the most important points you brought up was whether or not the success of Dr. *McCarty's* procedure is the result of surgical denervation or if it is due to some other factor. I would like to ask Dr. *McCarty* to respond to that point first.

*Dr. McCarty*

As far as the denervation being a factor, I agree, I don't think it matters what you do. You would probably get some effect over a period of time, perhaps a year, strictly from the denervation of the joint. But we have quite a few patients now who have gone four and five years with fairly good results. I am not saying they all work, because they all don't, but I feel that if the surgery is done correctly, and followed up with good occlusal stability, you are probably going to get a good result most of the time. Most of my patients are females, and I can't explain this either. Perhaps woman are just more prone to stretch injuries. As far as treating pain and clicking, I am treating strictly the pain, not the clicking. The clicking is but a parameter by which you can judge the success of your treatment.

As far as the validity of transcranial radiographs are concerned, I take that point very well. Apparently you all know a lot more about transcranial films than I do, but we have backed up quite a number of these with tomography and we still see the same thing. I believe this may depend upon who is taking the film, and I am not saying this for myself because I don't take the films; Dr. *Farrar* does all that. We found out for the most part that this is diagnostic for us, although I will agree that it shows strictly the lateral one half of the mandibular condyle.

*Dr. Solberg*

I would like Dr. *Petersson* to comment on the transcranial view since he did a Doctoral thesis on this topic.

*Dr. Arne Petersson* (Sweden)

We compared tomography and transcranial radiographs regarding condyle position and radiographic joint space. The transcranial radiographs are not reliable concerning the joint space, and they differ from tomography very often. If you want to see the joint space you have to rely on tomography.

*Dr. Hansson*

You know, we haven't seen so many anteriorly displaced discs in Sweden, and I was happy when Dr. *McCarty* explained it to me–that you have more orthodontists over here! Dr. *Solberg* made up some slides from our UCLA autopsy material that I think we should look at together. This slide is an obviously anteriorly displaced disc in a 31-year-old female. Almost all of the body of the disc is in front of the condylar head. In this frontal section from another specimen, the disc is medially displaced with a good deal of remodeling apparent, as well. I think that the surgery, itself, is fantastic, and I must say that we have to go home to Sweden and really look for these displaced discs.

*Dr. Blaschke*

We have looked at several hundred TMJ radiographic series at UCLA in the last few years. These series contain transcranial radiography and lateral corrected tomography and we can make comparisons on a day-to-day basis. Although I haven't done a study like Dr. *Petersson* has, it is my opinion, that the transcranial radiographs give a fairly true representation of the relationship of the condyle to the fossa. We have seen several cases where the tomogram will show the condyle concentrically placed in the fossa and the transcranial will make it look more posterior in the fossa. Therefore, if you are doing a scientific study on the spatial relationship of the normal joint, it is my opinion that tomography is the only way to go. On the other hand, if you are out in a busy private practice situation, then I think that transcranial radiography is very helpful and that you can depend on it most of the time.

*Dr. Mahan*

I just wanted to make a comment on Dr. *Laskin's* studies regarding the interpretation of transcranial radiographs. Weinberg published a paper showing this same thing a number of years ago. I, too, have done the same thing and it is clear that we are just looking at the lateral aspect, as you point out.

In most radiographs, except in children, the condyle has a kidney bean shape and you can usually see its outline in the transcranial radiograph. I think it is fine as long as we realize what we are looking at and I think most people today do recognize the limitations of this projection. Now it has been demonstrated that you can cut out a centimeter sphere of bone on the medial condyle and you can't see it because the X-rays are going down across the medial pole, and down across the neck and toward the film. As a result you see extra bone over the medial pole. What we need is an inexpensive way to look at the medial pole of the condyle. I think the transmaxillary view that Dr. *Öberg* showed yesterday will very often allow adequate visualization of the medial pole. I think we can get both the lateral and the medial with those views which I agree, are still secondary to tomography.

*Dr. Solberg*

There is one point I would like to look at a little closer. That is, we have been shown arthrograms and some histological specimens that show discs that appear to be thickened, yet there have been statements made that discs cannot proliferate or regenerate. I would direct this question to Dr. *Öberg* or Dr. *Moffett* and I would just ask, can discs proliferate, especially in the dense portion? Or if they do not proliferate, how can one explain the apparent change in disc dimensions?

*Dr. Moffett*

In the studies that we have done on monkeys with experimental disc lesions, I would say it depends on where the lesions are made. When we have made them in the centrally loaded avascular part of the disc and sacrificed the animals at lengthening intervals, I haven't seen the slightest sign of repair in that region. On the other hand, when we have made lesions of different types around the periphery of the disc in the vascularized, loose areolar connective tissue regions, frequently within two weeks after the time the experimental lesion is made one has difficulty identifying that this was the area in which we actually made a lesion. I think it's a question not so much of proliferation of the disc as perhaps a redistribution of tissues. There is some malleability in these structures, and I am not so sure that the change in shape takes place only by hypertrophy or hyperplasia because I can't demonstrate these processes in that loaded or central part of the disc. But it does seem that whenever an alteration in joint contours occurs, the disc seems to adapt to it quite well, not through this cellular process that I looked for and couldn't find but, rather, through some other unknown mechanism.

*Dr. Glenn Clark*

Dr. *McCarty,* you showed some of your slides where the disc was apparently deformed into a ball shape instead of the biconcave shape. With a patient who has chronic closed-locking, would you anticipate that the disc would be deformed so much that you could not reposition in surgically?

*Dr. McCarty*

You can only speculate how long the disc has been displaced. We see many discs that are either thickened or deformed into some unusual shape. You have a choice of what to do. If conservative therapy has been unsuccessful, then I think you have several choices. You can either take the disc out, or leave it in and attempt to repair it. You can do a condylectomy, or you can do nothing to the condyle whatsoever. It is my opinion that if it is possible to leave the disc in place, do a conservative recontouring of bone and attempt to relocate the disc. As a matter of fact, we have done quite a few total perforations and we were able to repair them. These have done rather well now, some of them going on four years.

# Concluding Remarks

Too often, TMJ disorders have been identified as disturbances of function, without due consideration to the structural alterations that according to biological laws, normally occur in association with dysfunction. For this reason, major attention has been focused on our emerging knowledge of TMJ intracapsular changes in this book. The resulting viewpoints of the contributors should have aroused an awareness among the readers of the significant role that intracapsular structural alterations play in the so-called TMJ (MPD) syndrome. It is also hoped that this book has been rewarding for those readers attempting to establish a more clear appreciation of abnormal joint morphology, including the existence and prevalence of soft tissue TMJ alterations. Our opinion is that this new knowledge will be of great value in overall patient management, in arthrography, in conventional radiography and in TMJ arthroplasty.

The contributors have also stressed the importance of developing specific diagnostic tests for identifying disorders of the TMJ and musculature. The contributors have given us some of the first evidence that quantifiable methods for identifying early TMJ lesions may be practical. With these new diagnostic techniques, prevention of serious problems is more desirable, but some forms of the structural derangements may be best treated by direct surgical intervention. Even with this knowledge, much remains to be known about the relationship of TMJ lesions to the unique pain and discomfort suffered by each patient.

As suggested by those contributors stressing the progressive nature of TMJ arthropathy, more has to be learned about the natural history of TMJ disease, without which no treatment will be well founded or predictable.

William K. Solberg
Glenn T. Clark

# Index

## D



## E



## F



## G

**M**



**N**



**O**



**P**

## R



## S

John W. McLean, O.B.E., D.Sc., M.D.S., L.D.S., R.C.S.

# The Science and Art of Dental Ceramics, Volumes I and II

In the first volume of this timely monograph, *The Nature of Dental Ceramics and Their Clinical Use,* the fundamentals of ceramics, including applications in jacket crowns and combinations with cast restorations are discussed along with therapeutic alternatives for the attainment of better, more esthetic results in those cases where conventional methods are insufficient to provide optimal results.

The second volume, *Bridge Design and Laboratory Procedures in Dental Ceramics,* presents detailed techniques for making metaloceramic and alumina-reinforced crowns and bridges. Such topics as special effects in dental porcelain, the "Wedge Technique," development of correct anatomy, methods for avoiding loss of detail during glazing, casting techniques, and surface finishing of metal are critically examined in light of recent research.

Vol. I: 336 pages; 229 illustrations (56 color); ISBN 0-931386-04-7 publ. 1979
Vol. II: 512 pages; 820 illustrations (680 color); ISBN 0-931386-11-X publ. 1980
Linen-bound with dust cover; 17.5 x 24.5 cm